We dedicate the two books we have written on how to incorporate isometric exercises into Nordic Walking and Trekking to Ian Northcott BEM.

Ian is an expert exercise coach, a great Nordic Walker, Trekker, and a man who has selflessly given outstanding service to his country and the community he lives in.

Isometric Exercises for Nordic Walking and Trekking™

Part 2. Exercises for Walk Partner-Pairs

Strength, Muscle and Stamina Building Exercises to Improve the Walking Experience and to Perform During Walking Breaks Anywhere

Published by

MajorVision International

2019

Approved by The World Isometric Exercise Association

www.TWiEA.com

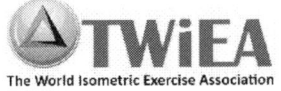

The World Isometric Exercise Association

Artwork, designed by MAJORVISION.COM

Contents

Important General Safety and Health Guidelines

This section entitled, "Important General Safety and Health Guidelines," pertains to The ISOfitness™ Exercise System, and all books and publications about it not limited to but including The ISO90™ Course, Fitness on the Move™, The 70 Second Difference™, The Bullworker Bible™, The Sixty Second Ass Workout™, The Bullworker 90™ Course, The Bullworker Compendium™, Workout at Work™, The Doorway to Strength™, TRISOmetrics™, The TRISO90™ Course, the TRISOmetric™ system, The ISOmetric Bible™, Isometric Power Exercises for Martial Arts™, Isometric Exercises for Nordic Walking and Trekking™ Part 1., and Part 2., general and specific recommendations, suggestions, coaching, and advice, either written, verbal, in audio format, on video, written, or given, implied, or suggested the authors, from Brian Sterling-Vete, Helen Renée Wuorio, and the works thereof.

You should never begin any kind of sport, exercise system, workout plan, or diet modification, including everything contained in this book and in any books mentioned in the beginning paragraph above unless you have consulted with and have the full approval of your medical doctor.

Your physician can properly assess your current health status, and your ability to perform the exercises in the book and/or course. This is particularly important if you have any known or unknown pre-existing health issues, if you're pregnant, or if you believe that you may have other serious health conditions.

It's essential that you must always have the absolute approval from your physician/GP before starting. Please show all the material in the above courses, books, video/audio, online material, and their content to your physician and get their approval before you start.

All exercises, suggestions, recommendations, instructions, exercise plans, dietary and eating recommendations, either given or implied, are intended only as a reference, and they are no substitute for a qualified professional personal coach who can help you to plan an exercise and diet program appropriate for your age and physical condition. Never overexert yourself when performing any exercise.

Stop exercising immediately and always either consult your doctor and/or call the EMS immediately if you ever experience any pain, irregular heartbeat, shortness of breath, tightness in your chest/arms/fingers, faintness, nausea, or feelings of dizziness.

The exercises, courses, plans, and dietary recommendations in this book together with all those mentioned in all the books, general publications, online material, and videos mentioned in the names in paragraph 1 of this section, are not intended for use by children. Keep all exercise equipment out of the reach of children.

Always inspect any exercise equipment, and/or any/all other improvised or specifically made exercise equipment/materials, doors, door jambs, and door frames, and anything else you use before each use to ensure its proper operation and to ensure that it is undamaged and safe. Do not use it unless all parts are free from wear, and it is functioning properly.

To avoid serious injury, care should always be taken using any/all exercise equipment, and in all items, people, books and courses, mentioned in paragraph 1 of this section.

Care should always be taken when getting into all exercise positions, on and off the floor, on and off chairs, on and off benches, on and off any other surface that might be used for exercise, including pieces of furniture, and in the use of all exercised equipment, either purpose-made or improvised.

The creators, writers, instructors, originators, and owners of The Bullworker90™ Course, The TRISO90™ Course, The ISO90™ Course, and all other courses/books, publications on video, audio, and in print, together with the courses, and websites, owned, originated, and created by the copyright holders and the ISOfitness™ and TWiEA™ team, including, but not limited to all books, courses, and people mentioned in paragraph 1 of this section, accept no responsibility whatsoever for any injury, harm, damage, illness, harm, damage to property, or any other negative health-related condition which may occur as a direct, or indirect result of following these courses, recommendations, suggestions, diagrams, pictures, videos, or while performing any exercises in these or any related other related material/publication/s.

For additional general information, we also recommend that you check reputable accredited medical advice sites such as the two listed here. The National Health Service in the United Kingdom, online at: https://www.nhs.uk/Livewell/fitness/pages/physical-activity-guidelines-for-adults.aspx

In the USA, The Mayo Clinic online:
http://www.mayoclinic.org/healthy-lifestyle/fitness/in-depth/exercise/art-20047414

Introductory Notes and Precautions

This book is one of two companion books, both called Isometric Exercises for Nordic Walking and Trekking™. The difference being that Part 1 focusses on different exercises than Part 2. However, both books detail the overall benefits of isometric exercise and how to perform isometric exercises to enhance the Nordic Walking and general Trekking experience and also exercises that can be performed during walking breaks outdoors.

The first book (Part 1) is entirely dedicated to exercises that can be performed as an individual, and the second book (Part 2) is entirely dedicated to exercises that can be performed in pairs as walk-partners, or walk partner-pairs as we call it.

The introductions to both books will contain either the same or virtually the same information. This is because the underlying exercise science of isometric exercises does not change, nor does the science about how muscle grows, and how fat is burned etc.

Both books contain sections of detailed information describing how to perform exercises that will target, strengthen, and tone all the main parts of the body. They also contain large descriptive pictures together with arrows that indicate the suggested direction which the exercise force should be applied. The exercises are not laid out in any kind of course format. Instead, the exercises are listed out to show what exercises can be performed for each body part so that individuals and fitness professionals can simply choose which of them they would like to perform according to their individual objectives.

Since both books contain all the essential information to exercise either individually, or with a walk-partner, if someone chose to read only one of them they would be fully prepared. This means that depending upon the objective, either book or both books can be used as a valuable stand-alone resource for use in the field by both Nordic Walking group leaders and for those who lead Trekking groups.

This shared introduction process for this topic also means that if someone already owns one book, then if they decide to buy the other, they have already ready the critical information about the exercise system and can go directly to the exercise section. However, we'd always recommend that everyone recaps the important health, safety and health guidelines every time.

Perhaps the most important benefit of all is that if the isometric exercises are practised regularly at home either as an individual or with a partner, then they will greatly improve one's overall strength, fitness, and endurance for both Nordic Walking and/or Trekking, and for life in general.

The exercises listed in this book, Part 2., are designed to be performed in conjunction with an exercise partner, so they will need to be adapted in order to be practised as an individual. Some exercises may not directly interchange so you will need to find alternative exercises for the same body part/muscle group.

Therefore, we suggest that if you wish to exercise at home using the highly effective isometric system, then it's best if you get a copy of Part 1, and/or The ISOmetric Bible™

(also available on Amazon) which is one of the most comprehensive and detailed isometric exercise books available today.

For more detailed information about fitness, healthy living, wellbeing, muscle and strength building, there is a list of other books about these subjects at the end of this one.

Special Precautions When Using Walking Poles

Remember, that when using walking poles as exercise tools one should always be extra cautious. Poles may inadvertently slip out of your hand/s at any time without notice, so be sure to take this into consideration and exercise with enough safety distance between you and anyone standing next to or generally near you.

Walking poles may slip on the ground without notice, so always be aware of this possibility and take precautions in advance just in case.

Also, many poles are constructed to expand by opening and closing screw joints along the length of the pole. Always ensure that these are firmly secured whenever the length of pole is adjusted and especially before all isometric and other exercise sessions which use the pole/s as an exercise tool.

Walking pole joints may fail at any time without notice, and no matter how unlikely this may be, one should always be aware of this possibility and be prepared for it. If in any doubt about the structural integrity of any kind of walking stick or pole, then do not use it for exercise or for any other purpose.

Chapter 1:
Nordic Walking and Trekking

We were first introduced to Nordic Walking and trekking by Ian Northcott BEM who is the founder of Mercian Nordic Walking in the UK. (https://merciannordicwalking.co.uk/)

Ian is a leading authority on all types of fitness training and the Chief instructor to TWiEA – The World Isometric Exercise Association. As well as being a thought leader when it comes to applied isometric exercise, Ian is a great believer in exercise being available for everyone and being able to exercise anywhere one chooses. This is completely aligned with our own concepts of exercise, and with our book called Fitness on the Move™.

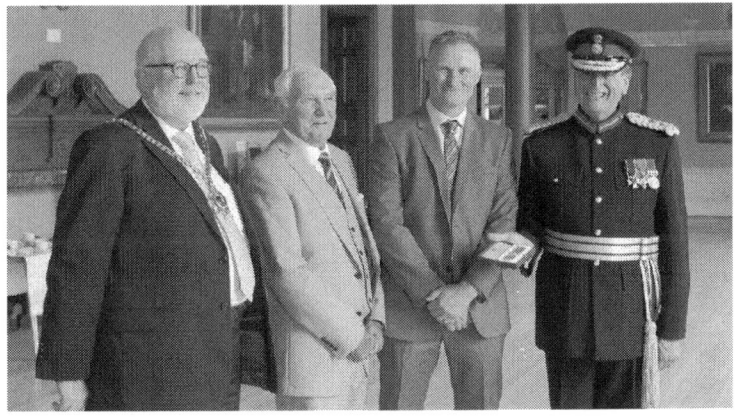

Ian Northcott BEM being presented with his medal.

Nordic Walking and general Trekking are both excellent forms of exercise that can be enjoyed by almost anyone of almost any age. Both systems offer significant health and fitness benefits for all who participate.

16

Nordic Walking, in particular, is an excellent total-body form of light general exercise because by virtue of the technique it employs it incorporates the use of many more muscles than regular Trekking with poles does.

If desired, Nordic Walking can also be performed in a much more strenuous way by athletes as a sport. However, for most people, Nordic Walking is simply a very healthy pastime which is often combined with pleasant social gatherings.

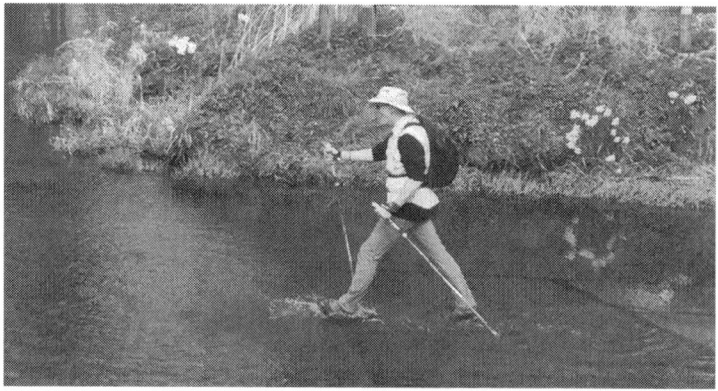

To greatly increase the health, fitness and strength-building benefits of Trekking and Nordic Walking, additional exercises can be performed during the regular break times enjoyed by most walkers and walking groups. An increasing number or walk leaders are now allocating time for specific improvised exercise sessions during walks with clients.

Perhaps the easiest and most effective form of exercise to engage in during a walking break is isometric. This is because it can be safely performed by almost anyone of any ages, it requires no special equipment while at the same time still delivering optimum results.

Also, it can easily be performed and enhanced by incorporating the use of Nordic Walking or Trekking poles as simple but highly effective isometric exercise tools.

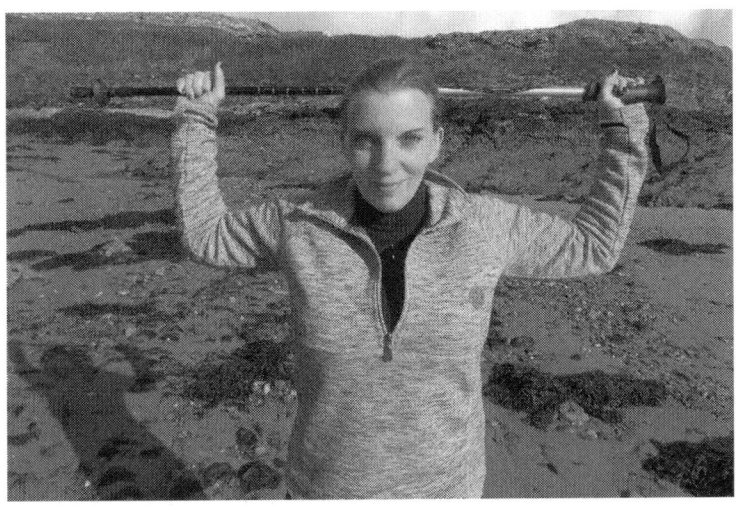

It should also be noted that isometric exercise is one of the most well-researched exercise techniques and has been proven to be superior to many other types of exercise when it comes to delivering maximum results for minimum effort in terms of muscle, fitness and general strength building.

Therefore, this is the exercise technique we will focus on. There is a growing number of Nordic Walking and general Trekking instructors who are specifically qualified and certified to teach isometric exercise to clients for use during walking breaks or at home.

More information about these instructors and how to find them can be found at TWiEA.com where a list of accredited isometric exercise instructors.

There is also information about how walk-leaders and fitness professionals can become qualified to teach isometric exercise should they wish to enhance the walking and fitness experience for their clients.

What is TWiEA™?

TWiEA™ is the acronym for The World Isometric Exercise Association which is the global governing body for all types of isometric exercise. TWiEA™'s mission is to help set and maintain standards of excellence in teaching and promoting all types of isometric exercise.

TWiEA™'s mission is to ensure that scientifically proven time-efficient isometric exercise techniques are taught to clients as part of an integrated overall approach to the total-body exercise solutions provided by fitness professionals. This creates a much higher probability that clients who are busy people, and who often face real-life time-crunches, can still maintain a regular highly effective exercise program.

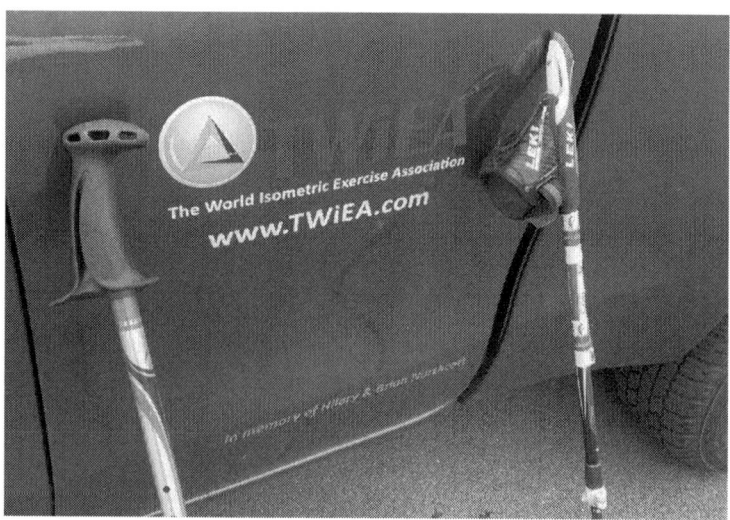

The fact is that isometric exercise is every bit as effective, and frequently more effective, at building muscle and strength as other more traditional forms of resistance training. It is also a timesaving and money-saving exercise solution that almost anyone can perform, even without equipment.

To begin with, and just in case anyone reading this book is completely new to Nordic Walking and how it differs from general Trekking with poles, I'll briefly describe what it is, how it works, and why it is different.

Nordic Walking Overview

Nordic Walking is very different to simply walking and Trekking while carrying general walking sticks or special walking poles. This is because in Nordic Walking many muscles of the upper body and core are engaged when applying force as the poles are deliberately engaged with the ground in a coordinated technique during each stride of a rhythmical cadence when walking.

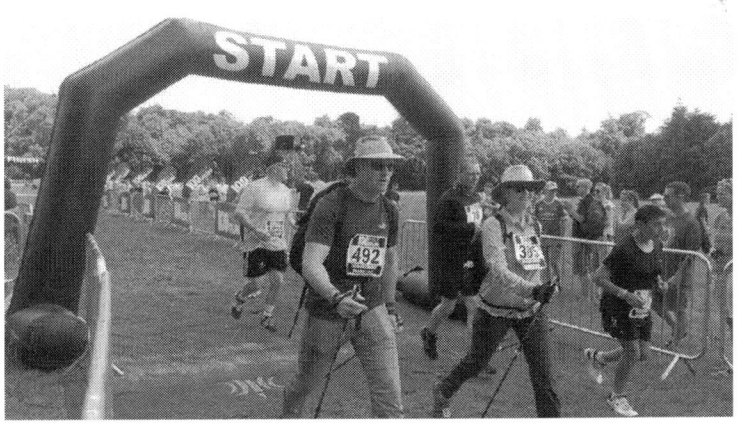

Ian Northcott BEM starting a Nordic Walking challenge.

In applying this technique, Nordic Walkers can apply as much intensity as is desired to all the muscles used during each stride. In turn, this gives the walker an enhanced fitness and strength building stimulus which regular walking and Trekking will not deliver.

The main muscles and muscle groups stimulated directly by Nordic Walking include the muscles of the rear upper back (Latissimus Dorsi), the chest (Pectorals), the shoulders, the triceps, the abdominals, the biceps, the forearms, and many of the core muscles.

In addition, the heart muscle receives significant stimulation when Nordic Walking at a reasonable pace, and it has been estimated that the technique produces up to 46% more energy consumption when compared to walking without poles in applied cadence with force.

The overall positive results produced by Nordic Walking are increased strength, flexibility, improved fitness and better overall coordination. There will also be other positive benefits gained in older adults in terms of maintaining bone density.

Trekking Overview

Naturally, Trekking is a form of hiking often incorporating the use of poles to provide some rhythm to a walking pace and for added support. On flat, smooth terrain poles aren't generally necessary although using them can increase the overall exercise value, as well as enjoying a general increase in overall walking speed.

However, on steep slopes, slippery rocks, and generally less certain terrain, poles provide increased lateral stability. Poles can also be used as aids when climbing rocks or boulders, to probe the depth of mud or water and facilitate a larger water crossing.

Nordic Walking Poles Overview

Nordic Walking poles typically feature a range of grips and wrist-straps, or on rare occasions, with no wrist-strap at all. The straps on Nordic Walking poles eliminate the need to tightly grasp the grips to help reduce overall fatigue on long walks.

Most Nordic Walking poles are made from lightweight aluminium, carbon fibre, or composite materials and they are significantly shorter than those recommended for cross-country skiing.

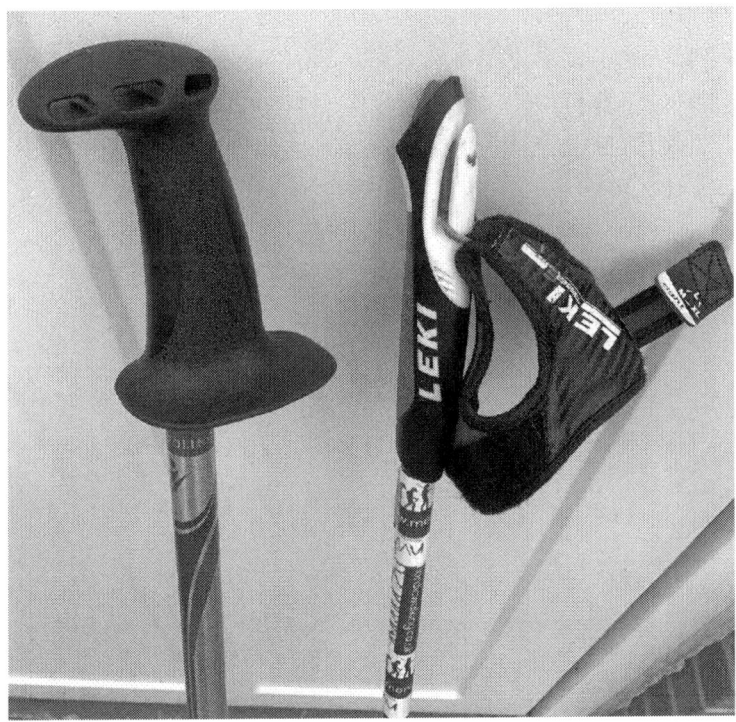

As with most Trekking poles, Nordic Walking poles incorporate removable/interchangeable tips, with rubber tips used on hard surfaces and hardened metal tips used on trails, beaches, snow and generally icy surfaces.

Nordic Walking poles are available in one-piece, non-adjustable shaft versions of varying lengths. These are generally the strongest and lightest, but this design has the obvious packing and stowage drawbacks.

Nordic Walking poles are also available in telescopic two, or three-piece twist-locking versions of adjustable length. These tend to be the most popular and adaptable.

Trekking Poles Overview

Trekking poles resemble ski poles and share many features in common, such as baskets at the bottom, rubber-padded handles and wrist straps.

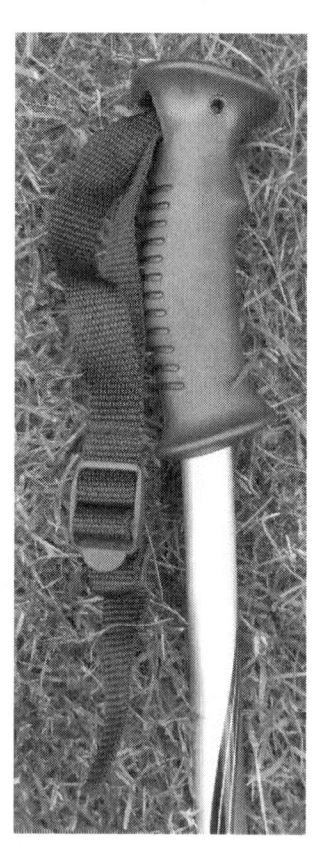

The maximum length of a Trekking pole is usually 135 cm (54 inches) which makes them adaptable for almost anyone of any age and they are usually made from lightweight aluminium or carbon fibre.

Unlike ski poles, Trekking poles are made in either two or typically three sections and can be extended and retracted as according to their use. This also means that they can easily be collapsed for easy transport and storage.

Some Trekking poles incorporate spring-loaded sections to aid walking under normal conditions and to reduce wrist strain.

The Choice of Poles in the Exercise Pictures

It should be noted that we deliberately chose to demonstrate the exercises in this book using standard Trekking poles and not Nordic Walking poles. This is because for exercise purposes they are essentially the same. However, since Trekking poles are much more common to find it is much more likely they will be used as IIED's or Improvised Isometric Exercise Tools.

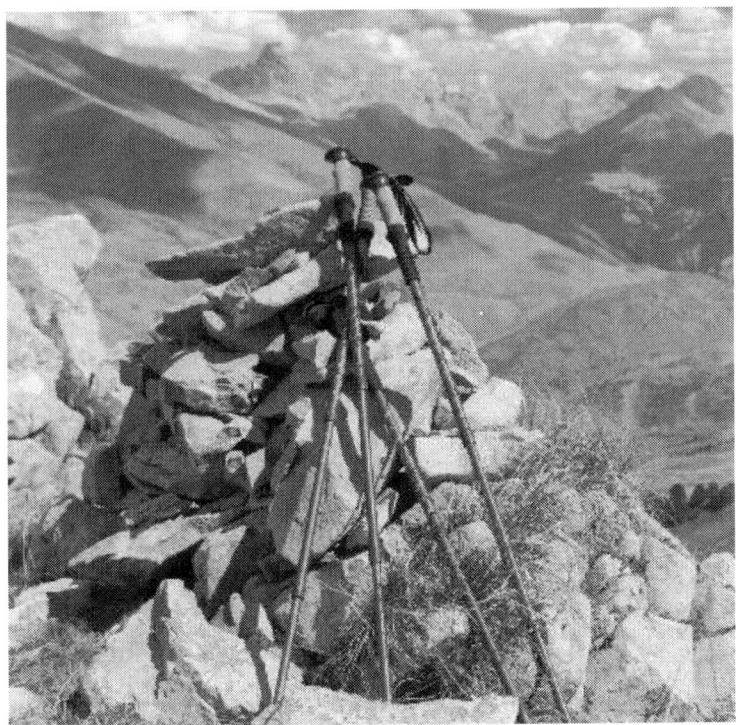

Chapter 2:
Exercise Science Overview

In this chapter, we'll give a user-friendly overview of exercise science together with the features and benefits of various exercise techniques and concepts. For those who want more in-depth information about the science of isometric exercise and health and fitness in general, then we suggest that you also read our books The ISOmetric Bible™ and The 70 Second Difference™ books. Both are available on Amazon.

Walking Vs Running as a Fat Burner

Walking and running are both an excellent way to get fitter, burn calories, tone up, and promote weight loss. There are different and distinct benefits to each which we'll briefly touch on. Running burns more calories than walking does. However, walking burns more fat than running does. So, it's a trade-off, especially since walking more will increase your N.E.A.T. factor. We'll explain more about N.E.A.T. in the next section.

When exercising at a lower intensity, fat is being used as the body's primary fuel. When you shift-gears and increase the pace from walking to running, then your body burns more carbohydrates as fuel. It doesn't really matter too much if you're burning body fat as the primary fuel, or if you're just burning carbohydrate as the primary fuel.

What is important is that you burn the most calories possible during your exercise session and stimulate a long-term increase in your Base Metabolic Rate. Therefore, even though walking may burn more stored fat as fuel, running will still burn more overall calories.

Another important factor to consider when looking at the differences between walking and running are the risks of injury from each. Running carries more risk of injury than walking, so the choice is yours.

Walking, General Activity and N.E.A.T. - Non-Exercise Activity Thermogenesis

The acronym: N.E.A.T. is becoming increasingly discussed in relation to weight control, body fat, and exercise. The N.E.A.T. acronym stands for Non-Exercise Activity Thermogenesis, and it comes from Dr James Levine's research into how we expend calories. In simple terms means it means: "burning calories through daily life, and not through exercise," and in very simple terms it means that people who are active and move around a lot, burn more calories and tend to be slimmer than people who don't.

There are two basic ways in which we burn calories. One is while we exercise, and the other is through the general activities of daily living. The key question is: "which, if any, is more important to weight loss, and the levels of body fat that we carry?" According to Dr Levine, it's the N.E.A.T. that appears to be far more important for calorie burning than dedicated exercise time. Dr Levine's research also led to the phrase: "Being Active Naturally" becoming more commonly used.

Providing that you're exercising good judgement in your food choices, and in the macros around proper portion control of your food, then in addition to your regular exercise routine, by just being a little more active in everyday life, it will make a huge difference in terms of weight control, and your overall level of body fat.

In our opinion, N.E.A.T. alone isn't a great panacea when it comes to losing weight and staying slim. After all, when people are stressed and mentally fatigued because of a tough workday, then it's not always easy to opt for the most sensible food choices, nor is it likely that you're going to want to go out and do something active to increase your daily movement factor. However, N.E.A.T. is certainly something to be factored into your overall lifestyle because it really does make a significant difference to your overall appearance and fitness levels.

The Basic Types of Resistance Exercise

All muscle training falls into between two or three specific categories, depending upon how you break them down. In the most basic form, there are two types, either contraction with movement, or contraction without movement. Breaking them down a step further there become three categories, with one being isotonic, another isokinetic. Last but certainly not the least, is isometric.

Isotonic training is all about movement with muscle shortening and lengthening during the lifting and lowering phases of the exercise. We know that the isotonic category can be broken down further into three parts.

One part being the concentric contraction, which is the lifting phase of an exercise when the muscles shorten in length. Another is the eccentric phase which is the lowering part of an exercise when the muscles lengthen. The last in this category is the isokinetic contraction. This is where the muscle changes in length during both the concentric and eccentric phases of the contraction, however, the velocity remains constant no matter how much force is applied during the exercises.

Finally, there is isometric training where there is no movement at all during an exercise. During an isometric exercise, a muscle is pitted against an immovable object or an opposing muscle/muscle group and placed under constant force for a set time. This is typically between 7 and 10 seconds for a standard isometric contraction.

Isometrics

As you now know, isometric exercise does not involve any movement. Instead, the joint angle and the muscle length do not change during contraction. Technically, 7 seconds is now regarded as the optimum time to perform an isometric exercise. However, since almost everyone when exercising tends to count the exercise elapsed time much faster than real elapsed time, 10 seconds is the target time most often used when people exercise isometrically.

Isometric exercise has been extensively scientifically researched and has been proven time and again to be a highly efficient way to build great strength and grow muscle. In fact, isometric exercise is probably one of the most thoroughly researched of all exercise systems. It also remains one of the most misunderstood systems of exercises. This is almost certainly through fear, professional ignorance and for purely financial reasons.

29

There are several different techniques that can be used in the isometric exercise system. Most of these techniques are highly advanced for use by competitive athletes, competitive martial arts practitioners, strength athletes and bodybuilders. Therefore, they have no application as part of a general isometric exercise session for the average person who simply wants to get generally stronger and fitter.

However, purely out of interest I'll list them here, and in case any fitness enthusiast, athletes or bodybuilders read this book and wish to try them. They are described in greater detail in our book called The Isometric Bible which is available on Amazon and good bookstores. The most common and advanced isometric exercise techniques include the following:

- ▲ Standard Isometric Contraction
- ▲ Yielding Isometric Contraction
- ▲ Maximum Duration Isometrics
- ▲ Oscillatory Isometrics
- ▲ Impact Absorption Isometrics
- ▲ Explosive Isometrics, AKA: Ballistic Isometrics
- ▲ Static-Dynamic Isometric
- ▲ Isometric Contrast
- ▲ Functional Isometrics
- ▲ TRISOmetrics™

There are more than enough isometric exercises that can be performed without any equipment whatsoever to allow a total body workout routine to be completed relatively easily. These will typically be self-resisted isometric exercises, which are excellent. However, by using only minimal readily available equipment such as walking poles, martial arts belts, climbing ropes, scuba diving webbing weight belts, and broom handles etc. it's possible to greatly expand the number of exercises that can be performed.

It's also perfectly possible to adapt and use other readily available items such as tow ropes, steel chains, towels, and commonly found immobile objects such as sturdy fixed barrier railings, solid walls, solid doors, door frames, or parked vehicles to perform a complete isometric exercise routine. Again, these are all excellent improvised exercise tools which allow an expanded range of highly effective isometric exercises to be performed.

Using improvised exercise tools can yield an unexpected additional benefit. This is that it allows one to focus more and apply greater concentration to each exercise. This is particularly useful for those who are either completely new to, or who are relatively new to the isometric exercise system. We'll explain more about what these can be later in the book.

One of the things we love about both the isometric and self-resisted system of exercise is that as you get stronger through exercise, then you can apply more force and intensity to your isometric or self-resisted exercises.

This, in turn, means that you can gradually increase the level of intensity you can safely apply to each exercise which will mean that the results and benefits you receive will grow in a compound way through regular daily use. This is what we call a natural Adaptive Response™ mechanism which is a very useful part of our biology.

Isometric Exercise Science

For those of you who would like to know more about the background and science behind isometric exercise, we'll briefly explain it now. Even until the mid-20th century, there was almost no scientific research that had been performed into the benefits of isometric exercise. We also know that prior to the first serious scientific research study, the way in which people trained isometrically was typically by performing what we now call endurance isometrics.

Thankfully, isometric exercise has now been thoroughly scientifically researched and proven for several decades. In fact, there has probably been at least as much scientific research performed into isometric exercise as there has into traditional resistance training.

The first major in-depth study into isometric exercise was performed at the world-famous Max Plank Institute in Dortmund, Germany. If you already have a reasonable knowledge of science, you'll also know that the Max Plank Institute is a world-renowned centre of scientific excellence in many disciplines. Between 1953 and 1958, one of the most extensive research studies was commissioned into isometric exercise science. These experiments are now considered by many to be the original "gold standard" of all isometric exercise studies. It was first made public knowledge in the resultant ground-breaking book, "The Physiology of Strength," by Dr Theodor Hettinger - Research Fellow at the Max Plank Institute.

During that 5-year research period, Dr Hettinger and Dr Muller performs over 5,500 experiments on volunteers from all walks of life, and at every level of strength, fitness and athletic ability. The test subjects even included serious strength athletes and middle-aged, overweight and unfit people of both sexes.

Perhaps what surprised people the most was how dramatic and impressive the results which were gained from performing isometric exercises. Also, because the same or extremely similar results were easily repeatable it made the data gained from the experiments very reliable.

The conclusion of the extensive studies proved beyond doubt the overall superiority of isometric exercise when it comes to building both strength and muscle, compared to traditional isotonic exercises methods. It also proved that the isometric system delivered these results much faster and with far less exercise than through traditional resistance training.

Another extremely interesting result emerged from the experiments. This was that it wasn't the length of time that an isometric exercise was held that produced the optimum results. Instead, it was the correct level of intensity applied for a specific optimum time.

They found that by performing only one daily isometric exercise for between only 6 and 7 seconds, and at only two-thirds of an individual's maximum effort, it had the ability to increase strength by an average of up to 5% per week. By any standards, strength gains of 5% in exchange for the expenditure of only 66%, or around two-thirds of an individual's maximum capacity, is an excellent result.

Perhaps even more amazingly, they discovered that after someone has performed a single 7-second training stimulus (exercise) per day, the muscle being exercised in that same position was no longer responsive to further gains. In other words, it didn't matter how many more times you exercised the same muscle in the same position, there would be no further increase in muscle growth or strength. The only way to do this was to perform another isometric exercise at a different position only the ROM (Range Of Motion) of the limb being exercised. The scientific data about this can be referenced on pages 28 to 31 of Dr Theodor Hettinger's book, "The Physiology of Strength."

In 2001, Nicolas Babault PhD of the University of Burgundy, Dijon, France, led a team of scientists to research and examine how many muscle fibres were activated, and how long they remained active for, during both traditional weight training and in isometric training.

(The scientific research paper is published: Nicolas Babault, Michel Pousson, Yves Ballay, and Jacques Van Hoecke - Groupe Analyse du Mouvement, Unite´ de Formation et de Recherche Sciences et Techniques des Activite´s Physiques et Sportives, Universite´ de Bourgogne, BP 27877, 21078 Dijon Cedex, France.)

They discovered that when training intensely, and in near-perfect style, the levels of muscle activation during repetitions of maximal weight training were between 89.7%, during the concentric contraction, or the lifting a weight, and 88.3% during the eccentric contraction, or the lowering of a weight. For practical purposes, an average of about 89% overall.

The study also revealed that during the lifting, or concentric, part of the exercise, the maximum intramuscular tension only lasted for between 0.25 and 0.5 seconds. Which, for practical purposes is an average of about 1/3rd of a second during each isotonic repetition. This is because traditional isotonic resistance exercises naturally involve movement. They also have aspects of velocity and acceleration to consider in the overall equation. "Force" is only produced for a split second, to produce a maximal contraction of the muscle fibres.

The same research also proved that the level of muscle activation during isometric exercise was as high as 95.2%, and that it lasted for the entire 7 to 10 second period of each exercise. The muscle activation also lasted for the 7 to 10 second period of the isometric exercise, which is a huge increase over the 1/3rd of second muscular activation achieved during a single repetition of weight training.

Therefore, based on these discoveries, then technically a single isometric exercise performed at only two-thirds of an individual's overall maximum can deliver either similar or often even better results, than the equivalent of up to 3 sets of 10 weight training repetitions in the lifting phase of the exercise.

To explain this further I'll use a typical barbell curl exercise as my example, where the object of the exercise is to engage as many muscle fibres possible in a maximum muscular contraction. Naturally, 3 sets of 10 repetitions give us an overall total of 30 repetitions. One set of 10 repetitions of the barbell curl in perfect high-intensity style produces a total maximum muscular engagement for a total of 3.3 seconds. Three sets of 10 repetitions of the same exercise, a total of 30 repetitions, this will give a total of 9.9 seconds of maximum muscular engagement, and an average of 89% muscle activation overall.

In comparison, if one high-intensity isometric contraction exercise produces a maximum muscular engagement that lasts for the entire duration of the exercise. Even though the optimum time over which an isometric exercise is performed was found to be 7 seconds, this is almost always rounded up to the 10-second mark. The maximum muscular engagement will last for the entire 10 seconds of a high-intensity isometric exercise and with 95.2% muscle activation overall.

This is proof that is based entirely on scientific research that 3 sets of 10 near-perfect high-intensity curls when weight training, which takes several minutes to perform, still wasn't quite equal to the results achieved by a single 10-second high-intensity isometric curl exercise.

The Standard Isometric Contraction

The standard isometric contraction is the exercise technique is simple and highly effective. Therefore, this is the technique we'll focus on for practical isometric training.

The standard isometric contraction, AKA: overcoming isometric contraction, AKA: maximum-effort isometrics, or whatever else you wish to call it, is when a muscle is applying force to push or pull against an immovable resistance. This is the most basic of all kinds of isometric exercise, and it's highly effective.

This type of isometric contraction exercise was performed during the experiments by Dr T. Hettinger and Dr E. Muller at the Max Plank Institute. It's also the isometric exercise technique referred to in their book "The Physiology of Strength".

In a standard isometric contraction, it is theoretically possible to exert up to 100% of one's maximum capacity effort against an immovable object and then continue to hold that level of intensity throughout the duration of the exercise. This means that standard isometric contraction can be a very high-intensity exercise system.

In performing an isometric exercise against an immovable object at a certain level of intensity for a given duration of time it will teach your body to recruit more muscle fibres to try to move the object. As you perform the exercise and generate as much force as possible, your CNS, or Central Nervous System, learns that it needs to activate and recruit more muscle fibres to reach the goal of moving the object. Since this will naturally be impossible to move, the process will continue each time you exercise to make you stronger and grow more muscle. This will also enable your body to more readily activate and recruit the extra muscle fibres as needed when a similar movement is performed dynamically.

Tas we mentioned earlier, the immovable/solid object that is used can be anything that is completely solid and completely safe to use. This can be a wall, a door, door jamb, parked motor vehicle or anything similar. Perhaps the most commonly used objects to enhance everyday isometric exercise training are sturdy towels, climbing rope, martial arts belts, scuba diving weight belts, webbing straps, Nordic Walking and Trekking poles, and broom handles, etc. All the aforementioned items are excellent when used properly, and all will deliver some excellent results. More importantly, they are typically readily available for most people which makes exercising with them so much easier.

Another common way to perform isometric exercise is to do it in a self-resisted way. Self-resisted means that you basically push or pull against your own limbs/hands/feet, etc. For example, you might place the palms of your hands together at chest level with your hands roughly at the midpoint of your body. In that position, you would then press your hands together using your chest muscles to provide the primary driving force. Suddenly, you're performing a very effective self-resisted isometric chest exercise!

It's possible to perform a very well balanced and highly effective self-resisted isometric workout to exercise virtually every section of the body. So, never underestimate self-resisted exercise because it can be very powerful indeed. In addition, self-resistance exercises are an excellent way to ensure that a personal maximum resistance is used safely, and with minimum risk of injury caused by applying too much force.

The fact is that it doesn't really matter which method is chosen. It can be isometrics performed against an immovable object, self-resisted isometrics, or a combination of the two. The most important thing is that either the object must be completely immovable through human muscle power alone, or the force of one body-part must be able to completely counterbalance the force of another body-part to produce a muscular stalemate.

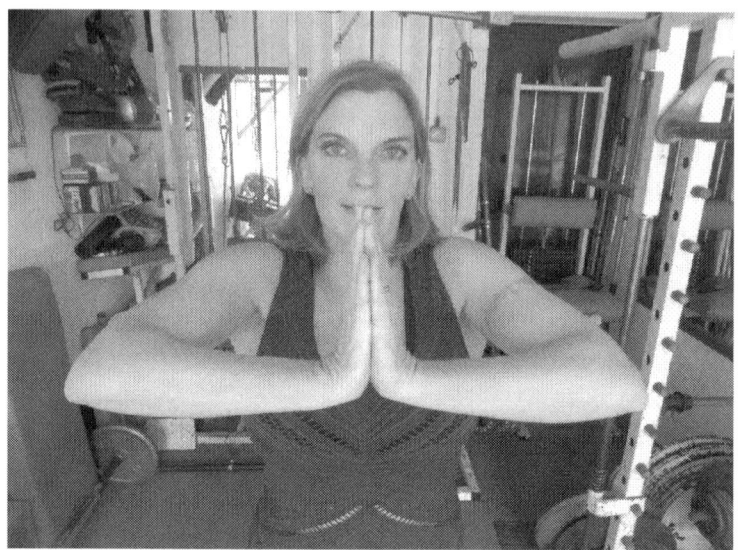

Workout Intensity

"Intensity" is always going to be a relative term, and it's often completely misunderstood when it's used in relation to exercise. Basically, when it comes to exercising your muscles, the intensity is the % of your ability to move a resistance. Technically, an individual's highest possible level of intensity is when they reach a point of momentary failure after exerting themselves completely.

However, the important questions we need to try and find answers to are: "How hard is hard?" and "How intense is intense?" To some degree, both are very subjective things. Taking two people of roughly equal

39

fitness, something that is intense to one person might be considered comparatively easy to the other.

"Hard" is a relative term, and even 50lbs of resistance is impossibly hard if your strength is only at the level required to lift 49lbs. However, if you're able to lift a 100lbs as a maximum, then lifting 50lbs is going to be comparatively easy.

Often, the only factors differentiating between people and the intensity level exerted, are going to be mental toughness, determination, and perception.

Therefore, in order to gain the greatest benefits from isometric exercise the first thing that must be learned is how to determine, with a reasonable degree of accuracy, what level of intensity is being applied to an exercise.

It's just a fact that what one person deems to be 100% of their capacity will always be very different from another person's estimate. The accurate estimation of what one person deems to be 2/3rds of their overall maximum intensity will also vary from person to person. The accuracy of estimation will also vary greatly between an experienced professional athlete and an absolute beginner to exercise.

Experience has taught us that most people who are new to exercise will always fall well short of accurate estimation of any given percentage. A beginner will find it more challenging to accurately estimate what 2/3rds of their 100% maximum is when compared to a more experienced athlete. Many people might believe that they're performing at 100% capacity when they're actually only performing at around only 2/3rds, or even perhaps at only 50% or less of their 100% maximum.

This is because exercise is new to them, therefore, the experiences and feelings in their body which are associated with it are also new. They simply have no common frame of reference when it comes to calculating/estimating their level of physical exertion.

The human brain has a built-in mechanism which helps to protect the body and prevent it from performing physical activity to such a level that could cause serious damage, or even death. This is the mechanism that makes your brain tell you to stop exercising when it begins to get tough, and the feeling of wanting to stop exercising only increases as you continue to push yourself harder to do more. This is all despite the biological fact that you're physically capable of doing much more than is being suggested by the messages you're receiving from yourself.

Over time, the brain of people who exercise regularly, and especially to a high level of intensity, will naturally adjust and reposition this built-in safety margin. This means that the brain of an experienced high-level athlete doesn't "tell" them to stop an exercise until the level of intensity is much higher than it would be for a beginner.

Therefore, when it comes to exercise, how is it possible to subjectively quantify, and then impart appropriate levels of recommended intensity? This problem is made even more challenging when one considers the fact that accurately translating and subjectively assessing various levels of intensity will, to some degree, always be subjective to every individual.

If you really do train as hard as humanly possible, with near 100% maximum intensity, which involves super-strict form, training to complete failure, and beyond, then you simply can't train for a long period of time. It's just physiologically impossible. Physics and biology are very simple in this respect.

The intensity of your workout is directly proportional to the length of time that you're physically able to perform your workout. The harder and more intensely you exercise, then the shorter time that you'll be physically able to perform the exercise.

Make no mistake, performing a 7-second isometric exercise while exerting close to your personal 100% maximum physical capacity is completely and utterly exhausting, even for a professional athlete.

What does all this mean when it comes to accurately communicate various levels of exercise intensity, especially when there's no professional coach or elaborate and expensive measuring equipment at hand?

Research clearly shows that almost everyone will stop exercising long before they're in any danger of becoming seriously fatigued. Most people will *"think"* they're achieving a much higher level of intensity than they would do if they were only a little more mentally resilient.

This doesn't mean that people should suddenly begin pushing themselves beyond their physical limits, which would be a stupid thing to do. However, it does mean that most people who enjoy a higher than average level of mental resilience and determination, as well as being in physically good condition, can push themselves much harder than they might think. If anyone ever feels "genuine" strain or fatigue to the point of becoming injured, then they should stop exercising immediately.

Even without the aid of a professional coach to monitor, encourage you and measure your intensity and progress with specialist equipment, the tips we've outlined in this section will help you to get the most out every workout. It's also worth remembering that if you cheat, then the only person who really loses every time is "you."

Technically, How Does Muscle Grow?

How does muscle grow? This is one of the most commonly asked questions in relation to fitness and exercise in general. However, it is also one of the most misunderstood concepts, even amongst fitness professionals and personal trainers. In order to see for yourself just how uninformed or badly informed some people are, simply join one or two of the social media groups online so you can read some of the absolute drivel posted by 'keyboard warriors' who purport to be 'experts' on the subject. Alarmingly, many of these people seem to have developed a hardcore following, which to the science-based professional is like watching 'fools leading other fools' on a wild goose chase.

So, back to the key question which is, how does muscle grow? To explain this, we must examine three concepts, which are: 1) muscle growth through increases in the volume/size of myofibrils inside the muscles, which is commonly termed as being myofibrillar hypertrophy. 2) hyperplasia, which is when there is an increase in the number of muscle cells/fibres. 3) sarcoplasmic growth which is all about increasing the fluid content.

When it comes to the subject of exercise, the muscles you wish to grow must be challenged with a workload which is greater than they can currently accommodate. In other words, exercise that is intense enough to stimulate growth. This stimulus can come from any source such as lifting a heavy object, weight training, isometrics, through compressing a spring in a device such as a Bullworker™, or through self-resistance either hand to hand / limb to limb / using an Iso-Bow™ etc.

This process creates trauma to the muscle fibres which disrupts the muscle cell organelles. This then triggers other cells outside the muscle fibres to greatly increase in numbers at and around the point of the trauma in order to repair the damage. The process of repair involves a fusion of cells. This, in turn, causes the cross-sectional area of the muscle fibre to increase because the muscle cell myofibrils increase in both size and quantity. This process is more commonly known as hypertrophy. Since this process increases the number of cellular nuclei the muscle fibres generate more myosin and actin. These are contractile protein myofilaments which in turn help to make the muscle stronger.

To summarize, this is the basis of what is more commonly known as myofibril muscle growth. In addition to this, there is also probably a process called hyperplasia which takes place. I use the term, 'probably' because this concept is extremely controversial for many reasons. One of the key problems being that evidence of this in human beings is lacking, whereas there is a mass of evidence supporting hyperplasia in mice and other animals.

Hypertrophy is the increase in the size of the existing muscle fibres to accommodate the increased demands placed upon them through intense exercise. Hyperplasia, with respect to skeletal muscle growth, is the increase in the number of muscle fibres which in turn will also increase the cross-sectional area of a muscle.

Despite there being a lack of evidence supporting hyperplasia in human beings, logic supports the process taking place. This is because of a theory known as Nuclear Domain Theory. This basically states that the nucleus of a cell (a muscle cell in this instance) is only able to control a finite area of cellular space. It is thought that satellite cells donate their nuclei to the muscle cell until a certain point is reached whereby this can no longer take place. Beyond a certain limit, and through continued intense training, the cell must eventually divide to create two cells instead of the former single cell. When this happens, the entire hypertrophy process starts over once again. This probably means that most of the muscle growth is almost certainly caused through hypertrophy, and a much smaller percentage can be attributed to hyperplasia at any given point in the muscle stimulus/growth process.

Finally, there is a subject of sarcoplasmic muscle growth to address. Sarcoplasmic muscle growth is the increase in the volume of sarcoplasmic fluid in the muscle cell. This is the fluid and energy resources surrounding the myofibrils in your muscles containing mostly glycogen together with other elements including creatine, ATP, and water etc.

To clarify, glycogen is simply a type of sugar that serves as a form of energy. It's deposited in bodily tissues as a store of carbohydrates, and it's the body's main form of storage for the sugar, glucose. Glycogen is stored in two main places in the body, one being the liver, and the other being the muscles.

More importantly, glycogen is the body's secondary source of long-term energy storage, with the primary energy storage source being fat. When glycogen is in the muscles, it is converted into glucose for use as energy when performing sports etc., and glycogen stored in the liver is converted into glucose for use as energy throughout the body, and in the central nervous system.

Therefore, sarcoplasmic growth increases the muscle volume, but this increase is not in functional strength mass since it doesn't increase the number of muscle fibres. It's like 'the pump', in that it is an increase in the size and shape of the muscle through the muscle holding an increased amount of fluid.

Rest and Recovery

For those who have already read about this subject in "The 70 Second Difference™" book, they will know that rest and recovery after intense exercise is essential. This is because both your body and your immune system must be given sufficient time to recuperate properly.

If it's your intention to significantly increase your muscle size and strength, then it's always worth remembering that your muscles don't grow during your workout. The workout phase is the stimulus, and the real growth process begins after your workout is over, during the recovery period.

Exercising too often will prevent complete recovery from taking place, and it will eventually deplete your muscle tissue. It will have the completely opposite effect to what you wish to achieve.

When calculating your ideal recovery period, many things must be taking into consideration. These include your age, your current health and fitness level, the quantity of exercise taken, and most importantly the intensity of the exercise which has been performed.

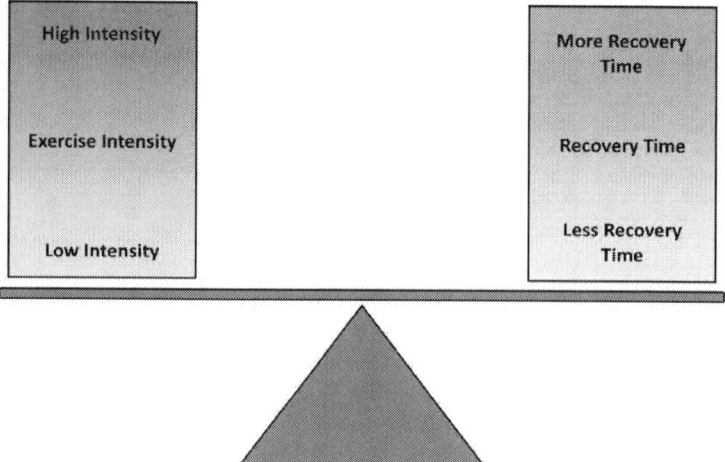

Some people will need a recovery period of between 24 and 48 hours, and for others, the recovery period may be as brief as between 12 and 24 hours.

As a rule, the recovery period will always incrementally increase as the intensity of the exercises increases towards an individual's 100% potential maximum capacity. Always be aware of this and make sure that you factor this into your rest and recovery time calculations. The following visual will help to outline this.

Sports scientist J. Atha's research revealed something remarkable. This was that when performing isometric contraction exercises at two-thirds of an individual's maximum capacity, the average person could safely perform an exercise like this daily, without overtraining.

Standard isometric contraction exercises can be safely performed daily, by almost anyone, of almost any age, and in almost any physical condition as a means of strength development, body shaping, and even for bodybuilding.

However, for workouts that are more intense, then we recommend a full rest day between workouts due to the higher demands being placed upon the Central Nervous System (CNS) and the time needed to fully recover and benefit from the exercise.

There are several other factors which affect post-exercise recovery. These include a balanced and properly executed stretching routine and getting enough quality sleep. While you sleep, your body releases certain hormones which help you to repair and rebuild damaged tissue, and which will directly help your muscles to grow.

Post-exercise high-quality nutrition will help your body to repair itself faster, decrease your recovery time, and will help to generally maximise the benefits gained from the exercise. Studies indicate that there is a 30 to 60-minute time-window after exercise when you need to eat, and after which, your body begins to draw upon itself to repair and recover from your exercise session. Drinking enough water is also one of the most important factors in your recovery, as well as for your overall health. This is because your muscles are mostly composed of water.

Rest Time Between Exercises

Naturally, the rest time taken between exercises during a workout is very different from the rest and recovery needed to recover and allow your body to positively respond to the stimulus generated by exercise.

If you keep the rest time between exercises brief enough, then the workout routine itself will give you an excellent cardiovascular workout, and this is what we recommend that you ultimately aim for. If you're already very fit, then we'd recommend that instead of performing the optional cardio routine, and you simply put more effort and intensity into each isometric exercise. At the same time, aim to keep the rest time between those exercises as brief as possible. This approach will help you work towards being able to perform each exercise so that it has an Ultra-High Intensity Ultra-Short Burst™ effect, which will greatly improve your overall fitness level, and boost your Base Metabolic Rate or BMR.

However, if you're not already fit, then to begin with you may wish to simply allow each isometric exercise to deliver all the cardio you need as you gradually build up your levels of fitness and endurance. Eventually, you'll soon increase your level of fitness to a point where you can begin to gradually reduce the rest time between each exercise to a minimum point that works best for you.

Once you've learned how to fully engage the muscles during each exercise with sufficient intensity, and at the same time you've learned how to breathe fully, deeply, and naturally throughout each exercise, while at the same time keeping the rest time between exercises to a minimum, then this combination will have an excellent and beneficial cardiovascular effect.

Dynamic Flexation™

Dynamic Flexation™ is a technique we devised to help ensure that we gained maximum benefit from the isometric portion of our own exercise regimens. Since we outlined it in our first publication, it has always been included in some form or another in all our books about ISOfitness™. I'll recap and briefly summarise the Dynamic Flexation™ technique as originally laid out in "The 70 Second Difference™" book.

Even for a beginner, we would always recommend that to some degree everyone employs a form of Dynamic Flexation™ before performing any exercise. This will help to ensure that all muscles, tendons, ligaments, joints, and your spine have become naturally and properly engaged in the correct biomechanical exercise position.

This is because when you are in a good position it will help you to gain the maximum benefit from each exercise you perform. Dynamic Flexation™ is when you move and adjust either your feet, legs/leg, hips and especially your hands as you gradually assume a solid position and handgrip. As you flex and move, you'll be making micro-adjustments.

Typically, all exercises will be performed best if you assume a correct handgrip, fist clench, or foot position etc. One of the most important aspects of assuming the correct exercise position begins with your grip. Without a solid grip on a bar, handle or anything else you need to hold while exercising, you'll naturally be setting yourself up to perform sub-maximally. You can also be helping to develop injuries which can include sore elbows, joints, ligaments and tendons.

When you begin to employ Dynamic Flexation™, initially, when you assume the correct exercise position you should apply almost no tension whatsoever. Instead, you should "feel" your way into ensuring that you're in the correct position. Only then should you begin to apply any tension to the exercise.

We'd never recommend that as soon as you assume an exercise position that you suddenly apply maximum power and intensity right away. This is unless you're a very experienced athlete, or unless you're training with a qualified coach to perform a certain type of isometric exercise to develop extra power such as a static-dynamic or explosive/ballistic isometric technique. Instead, we recommend that you always breathe naturally as you gradually flex and engage your muscles and joints into the exercise.

Our preference is to apply tension and intensity to the exercise gradually through Dynamic Flexation™ over a period of typically between 2 and 3 seconds, or even for as long as 4 seconds if needed. This all takes place before beginning to count the required 7-second exercise hold time of the isometric contraction.

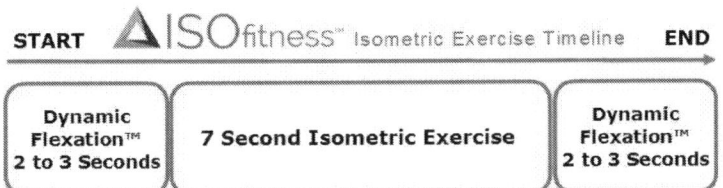

We prefer using one deep full breath in and out as a method of more accurately counting each second that has elapsed. This way, you'll time each exercise more accurately, and you'll not be tempted to hold your breath at any point which is a mistake that beginners often make.

Similarly, at the end of an exercise, we don't recommend that it be ended abruptly. Instead, we recommend reversing the Dynamic Flexation™ technique so that you gradually relax as you slightly move each muscle and joint out of the exercise position.

Dynamic Flexation™ is a concept which embraces the broader principles of motor unit recruitment, and "Henneman's Size Principle" to increase the contractile strength of a muscle. Elwood Henneman's principle stated that under load, the motor units in a muscle are engaged according to their magnitude of force output, from the smallest to the largest, and in task-appropriate order.

This means that the slow-twitch, low-force, fatigue-resistant muscle fibres are activated before any fast-twitch, high-force muscle fibres are engaged which are less fatigue-resistant. Since the body naturally works in this way, it

52

enables precise, finely controlled force to be delivered at all levels of output.

This also means that when exercising, or when performing tasks in daily life, the fatigue which is experienced as a result will be always be minimised. It will also be proportional to the sequential engagement of the most appropriate muscle fibres being engaged.

Isometric Exercises and Blood Pressure

Some exercise critics point out the fact that when someone performs an isometric exercise it will raise their blood pressure. However, the same people also very conveniently forget that the same is also true of all other forms of exercise including freehand callisthenics and traditional isotonic resistance training with weights.

ALL physical activity, and especially exercise will cause your blood pressure to rise for a short time. Providing that you are in good health, that you always breathe deeply, naturally and normally when performing any exercise, then any rise in blood pressure will soon return to a normal level when the exercise is stopped. The faster this happens, the fitter you are.

For those who are advanced athletes and/or are used to hard and intense isometric training for a long time, then you'll already have made significant progress in strengthening your heart and circulatory system.

For those who are new to isometric training, just like with any form of exercise, the best way into it is by taking it slowly and less intensely at first.

Newcomers to exercise, and especially isometrics, should always focus on applying less intensity, to begin with, and on always breathing fully and deeply throughout all exercises. NEVER HOLD YOUR BREATH!

Under strict medical supervision, even those with Coronary Artery Disease and high blood pressure should be able to increase their physical activity levels with a reasonable degree of safety safely.

However, if you're a person who already suffers from high blood pressure, then you should always exercise at a much lower level of intensity than someone who has no physical issues.

Furthermore, **EVERYONE, AND ESPECIALLY PEOPLE WITH HYPERTENSION, OR ANY FORM OF CARDIOVASCULAR DISEASE, SHOULD ALWAYS CHECK WITH THEIR DOCTOR BEFORE BEGINNING ANY KIND OF EXERCISE ROUTINE**.

Chapter 3:
Proprietary Isometric Exercise Equipment

We highly recommend and endorse the Iso-Bow®. as an exercise tool. This inexpensive little device is an amazingly versatile device that allows self-resisted isometric exercises to be performed very easily. It also allows self-resisted isotonic and what I call functional isokinetic exercises to be performed easily. The Iso-Bow® provides the user with a biomechanically sound grip handle which allows almost all exercises to be performed more effectively, and with greater ease and comfort.

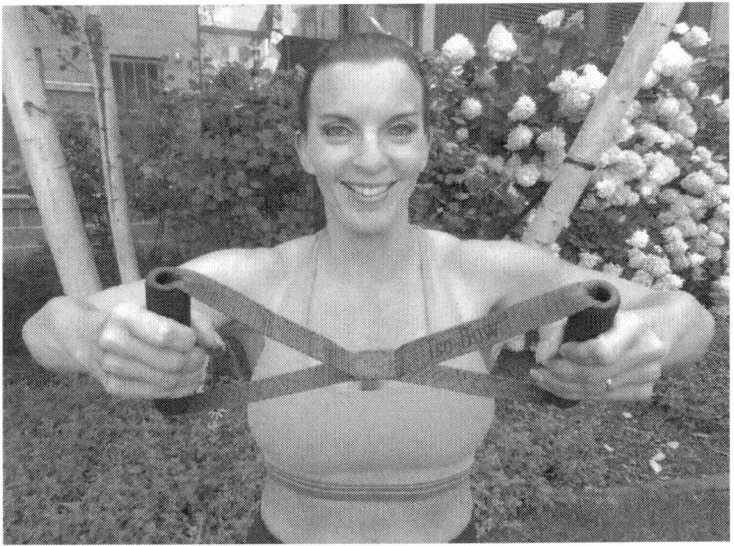

With a pair of Iso-Bows®, you can effectively exercise every major muscle group of the body, and even perform advanced exercises such as the pull-up, the squat and the deadlift. The level of workout you can get from using a pair of Iso-Bows® can range from an easy low-level beginner's workout, right up to a very high-intensity professional athlete level of workout. Amazingly, you can do all of this without any adjustment being needed to the Iso-Bows®. Each user will benefit proportionately, according to the amount of effort and intensity that is applied during each exercise.

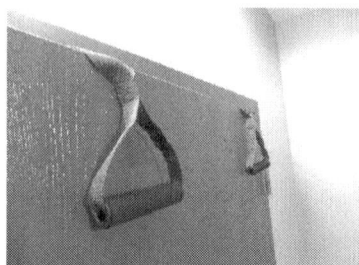 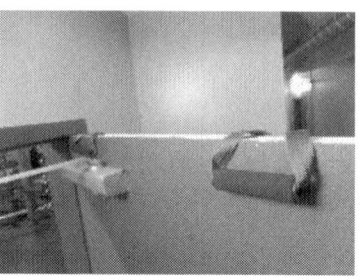

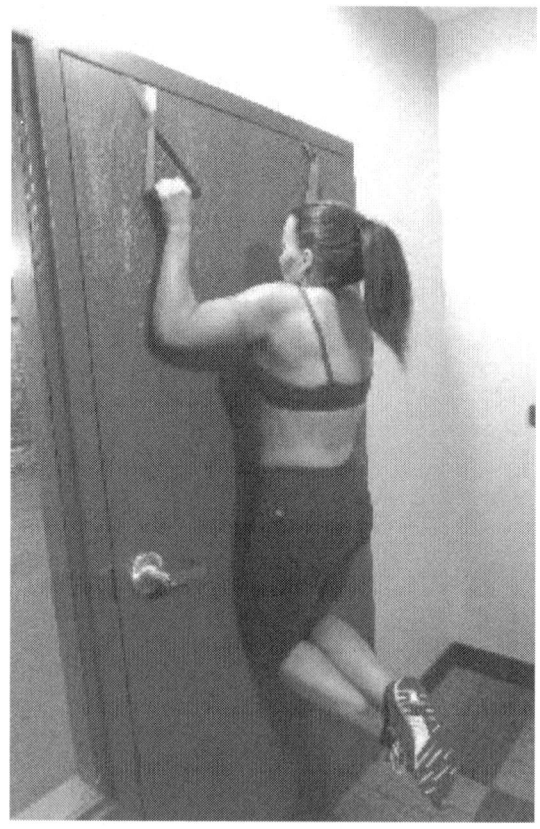

Even a pair of Iso-Bows® are so compact they can easily fit into the average jacket or jeans pocket, a small handbag/purse, a briefcase, or a walking rucksack or bag.

Perhaps the best-known of all isometric/isotonic home exercise devices is the Bullworker® which has been a best-seller when it was launched in the early 1960s. Today, it is still a best-selling device, and with good reason, because it really works. The smaller "partner" device is called the Steel Bow®, and both have interchangeable springe so that both men and women of all strength levels and abilities can use them, with roughly equal effectiveness.

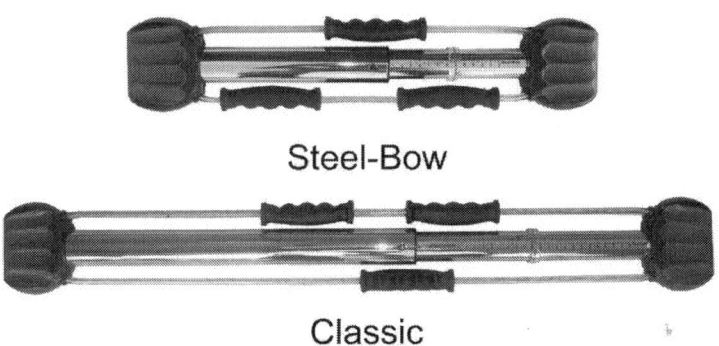

Steel-Bow

Classic

Securing the Iso-Bow® With Your Feet

When performing leg exercises such as squats and lunges, as well as lower back and glute exercises such as the deadlift, it becomes necessary to properly secure the Iso-Bow® using your feet. There are several ways in which the Iso-Bow® can be secured using your feet, and your personal preference of how you do this will depend upon many factors such as your foot size, your choice of footwear, and ease of operation.

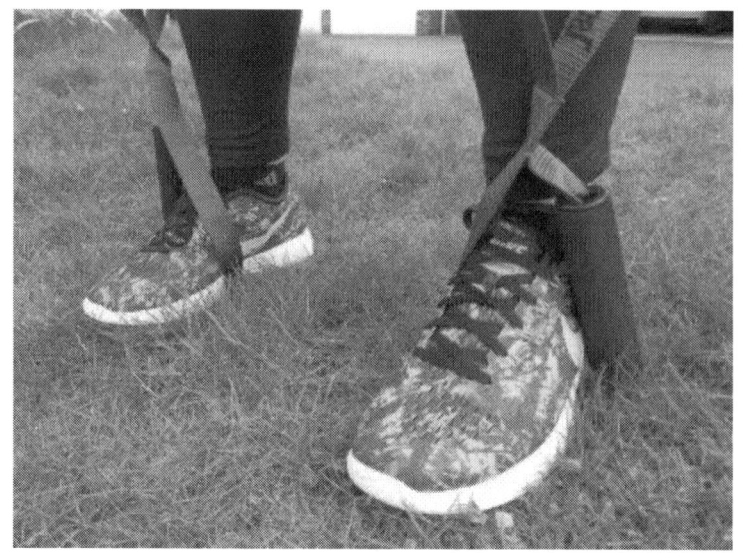

You can secure the Iso-Bow® with your foot inside one of the handles. You do this by adjusting the handgrip to one side, usually the outer side of the foot, and then place your feet inside the loop like a stirrup.

Another method is to place the Iso-Bow® flat on the floor and then stand on one side of the straps so that the handle of the same side sits flush to your inner foot. In this position, it will be your bodyweight combined with the handle pressing against

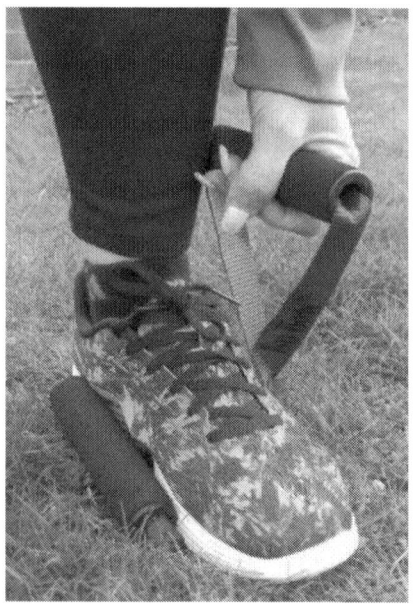

the inner side of your foot which enables you to pull safely and securely.

The final method is to simply place each foot through one end of an Iso-Bow®, stepping onto the foam hand grip as you do so. This method is slightly less stable than the other two methods.

However, if the foot can be pushed far enough through the loop of the Iso-Bow® handle, then the handle will slightly raise the level of your heel making it easier for some people to squat or lunge.

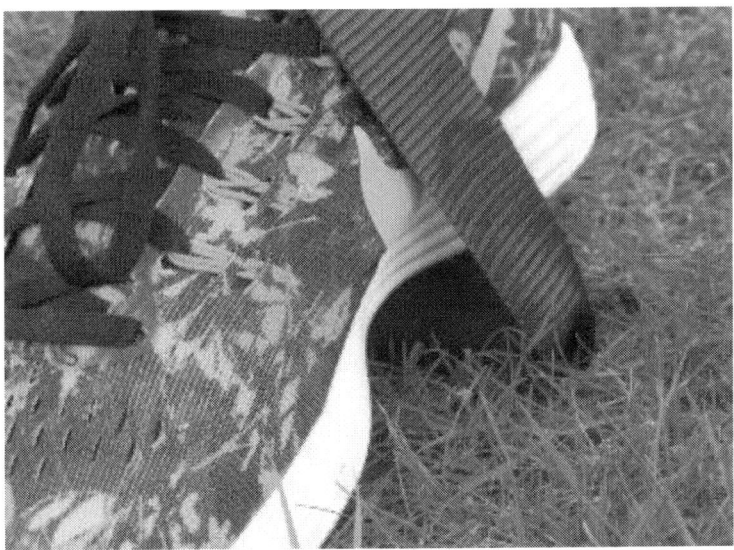

Naturally, safety is always a top priority so whichever method you ultimately choose to use, you should always make sure that when securing the Iso-Bow® with your feet that there is never any chance of it slipping in any way while you exercise.

Chapter 4:
Things to Remember Before You Begin

⚠ The first and perhaps the most important thing to remember is: **NEVER HOLD YOUR BREATH AT ANY TIME.**

⚠ Breathing in and out naturally during all isometric exercises will also help you count the number of elapsed seconds much more accurately, with one full breath in and out taking approximately one second.

⚠ We recommend that you read the instructions about each exercise carefully. You can also watch the associated videos via the TWiEA™ website if you wish to become a member and access the resource.

⚠ Remember to leave a safe distance between you and anyone near you when exercising with Trekking or Nordic Walking Poles.

⚠ Always check the structural integrity of Trekking, Nordic Walking, or any other type of improvised isometric exercise device. If there is any doubt about the structural integrity, then do not use it for exercise or any other purpose.

⚠ Double-check that all adjustable joints on Trekking and Nordic Walking Poles are secure before use.

⚠ Weight loss/fat loss will ONLY occur when any exercise plan is used in conjunction with a calorie-controlled diet.

⚠ It's critically important to completely focus your mind on the exercise being performed. In addition to this, it's important to envision the muscle that is being exercised is growing larger and stronger.

62

△ Always consult a professional coach to devise a detailed stretching routine, this will ensure that you're stretching the areas effectively rather than risking injury.

△ Always ensure that a stable line of biomechanical progression is achieved before engaging in and performing any exercise.

△ Warming-up, stretching, and cooling down are three of the most overlooked yet essential elements to exercise, and we cannot stress their importance strongly enough.

△ During ANY form of physical exercise, including isometrics, if you apply too much intensity too soon, then you may inadvertently strain a muscle. Isometric exercise is particularly intense, and a single isometric exercise engages a great many more muscle fibres than even high-intensity weight training, and isometrics engages the muscle fibres at a much higher level too.

△ When exercising in partner-pairs, extra caution is always needed. If one is totally reliant on a partner during certain exercises, if they accidentally or inadvertently slip or move it may cause you to lose balance, slip, lose good exercise style or even fall. Therefore, always be aware that this may happen, however unlikely it might be we suggest that you plan ahead to compensate for it.

△ Sometimes when exercising in partner-pairs, the partner who is supporting the exerciser should always try to stay one step ahead and anticipate any compensatory adjustments to balance or positions that may be needed in order to allow your partner to complete the exercise correctly. No matter how minor an adjustment to balance or position might appear on the surface, it may have a serious repercussive effect in it is not planned for and practised in advance.

⚠ When intending to workout with an exercise partner it's always advisable to practice the exercises with them in advance before applying your maximum desired exercise intensity.

⚠ When exercising in partner-pairs it's typically recommended that after one of the partners has completed an exercise, the other partner then performs the same exercise. This process should be repeated until the workout session has been completed.

⚠ In many of the exercises, the supposed assisting partner is also gaining an exercise benefit, so they should prepare and adapt themselves for this.

Therefore, for safety's sake, we're adamant that you should always gradually and progressively engage your muscles into ANY isometric exercise, and according to what we call The ISOfitness Exercise Timeline™.

The main benefit to properly warming up for several minutes before a workout is injury prevention, and to increase your heart rate and the circulation to your muscles, ligaments and tendons. It's important to remember that warming-up and stretching are two different concepts and that stretching isn't a good warm-up. This is because stretching will put the muscle in an un-contracted position and weaken it. Stretching is always best performed after a workout has been completed, together with a proper cool-down. In addition to properly warming-up, always perform a gentle "flex and stretch" of the muscles and joints which are about to be exercised. For example, squatting down fully to flex the thighs and loosen the knees is always a good idea before performing any leg exercises. Dynamic Flexation™ should always be used with every ISOfitness™ style isometric exercise. Here's a diagram which explains the workflow visually.

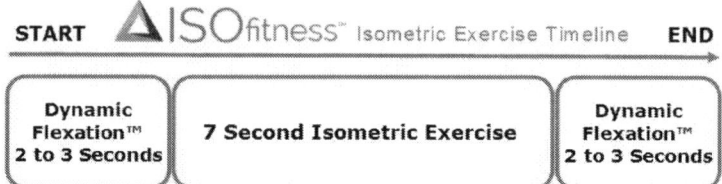

Chapter 5: About the Exercise Models

Helen Renée is the model in the section describing the exercises and how to perform them. Helen is a contest-winning bodybuilder and Bikini Fitness Competitor who exercises religiously every day, no matter where she is or where she's travelling to. Helen is particularly strong with the exceptional power-to-weight ratio one would expect from a former gymnast. She is also an isometric and TRISOmetric™ exercise expert instructor and instructor-trainer for TWiEA™ The World Isometric Exercise Association. www.TWiEA.com – www.HelenRenee.com

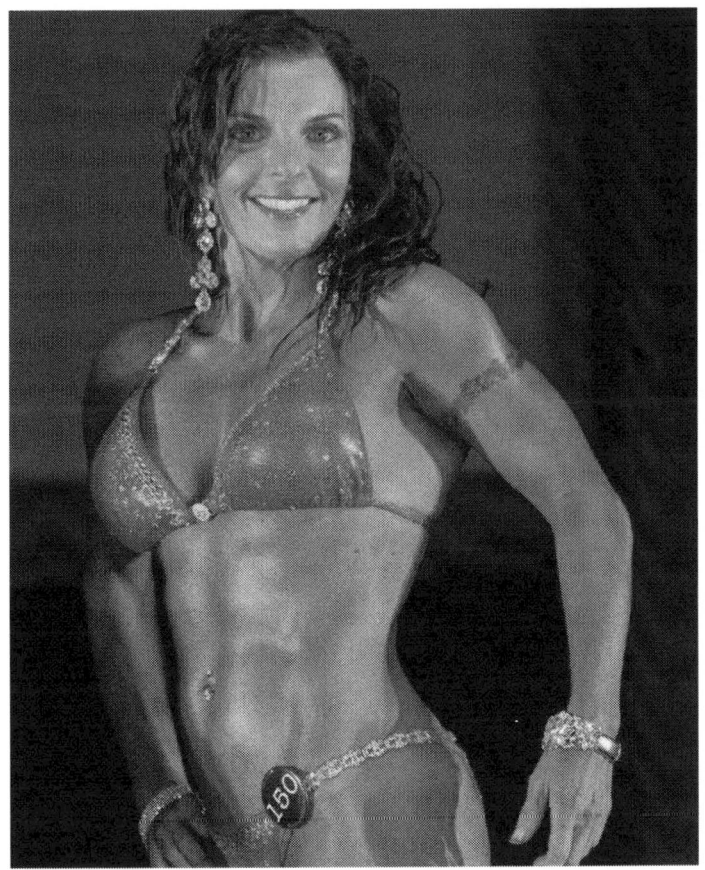

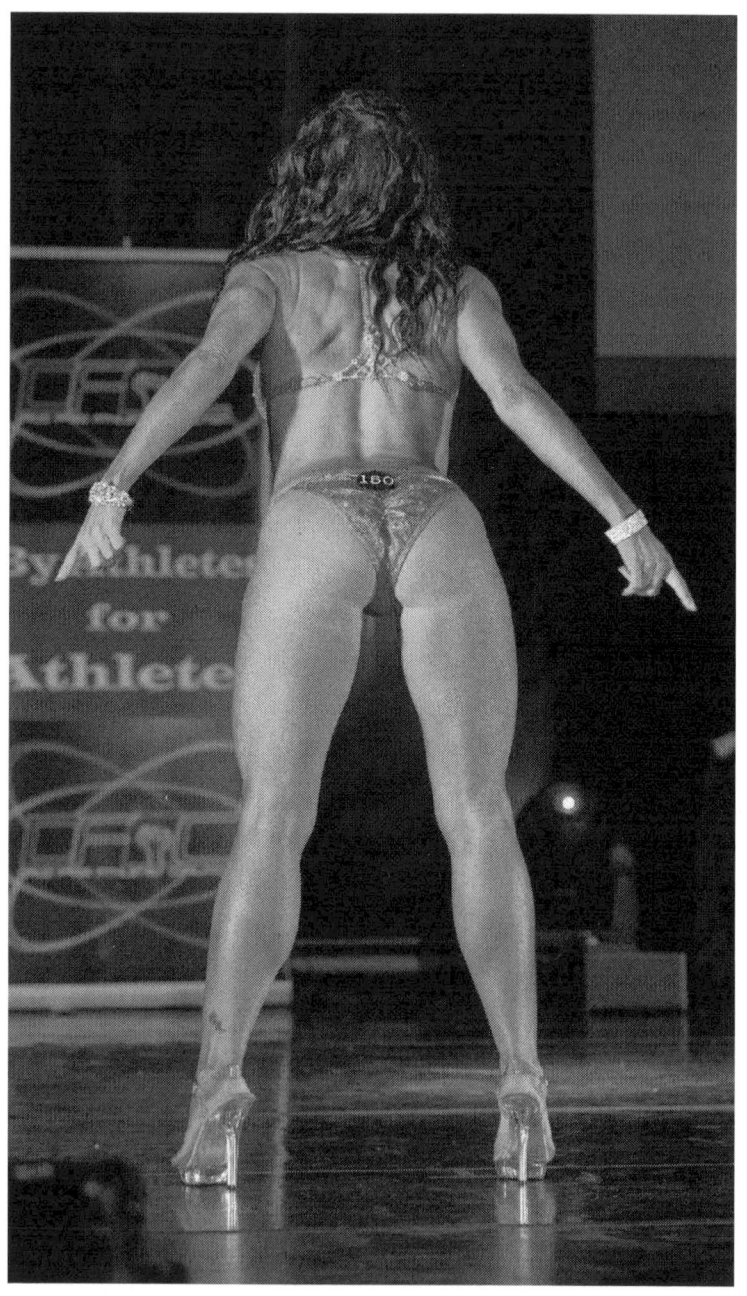

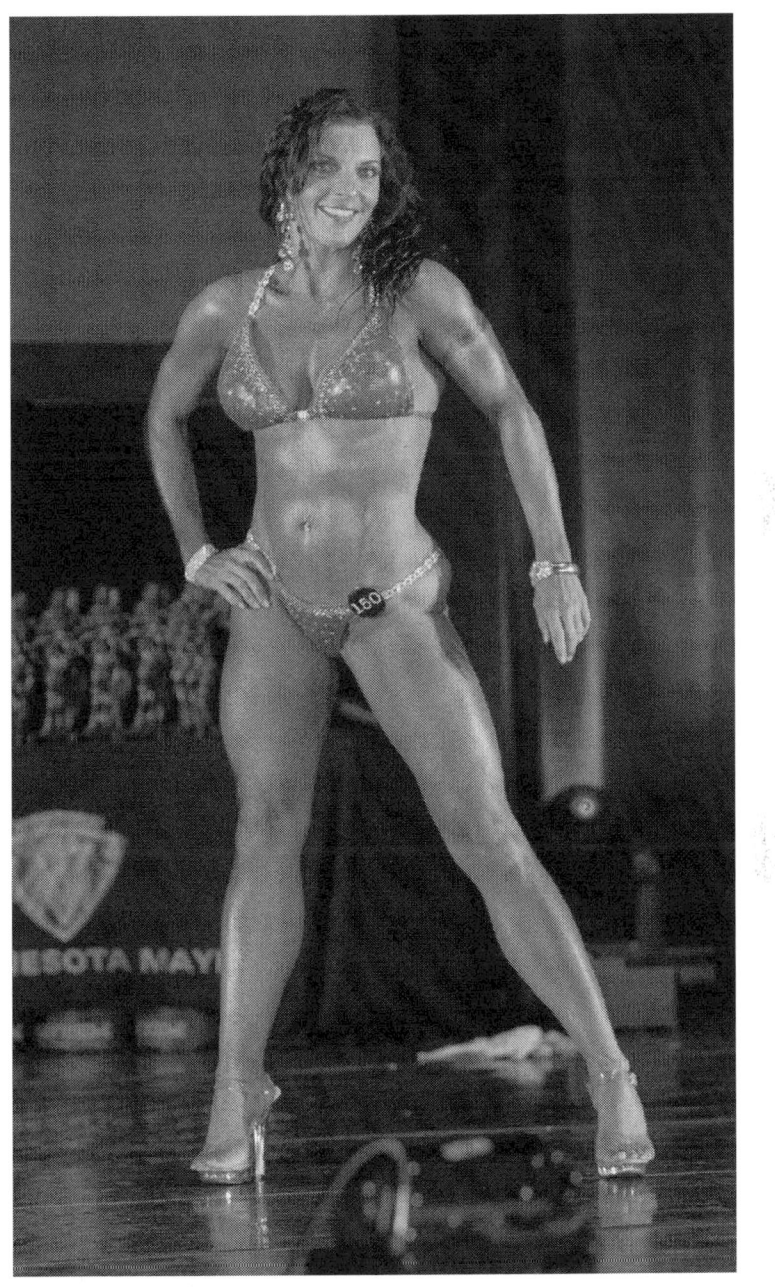

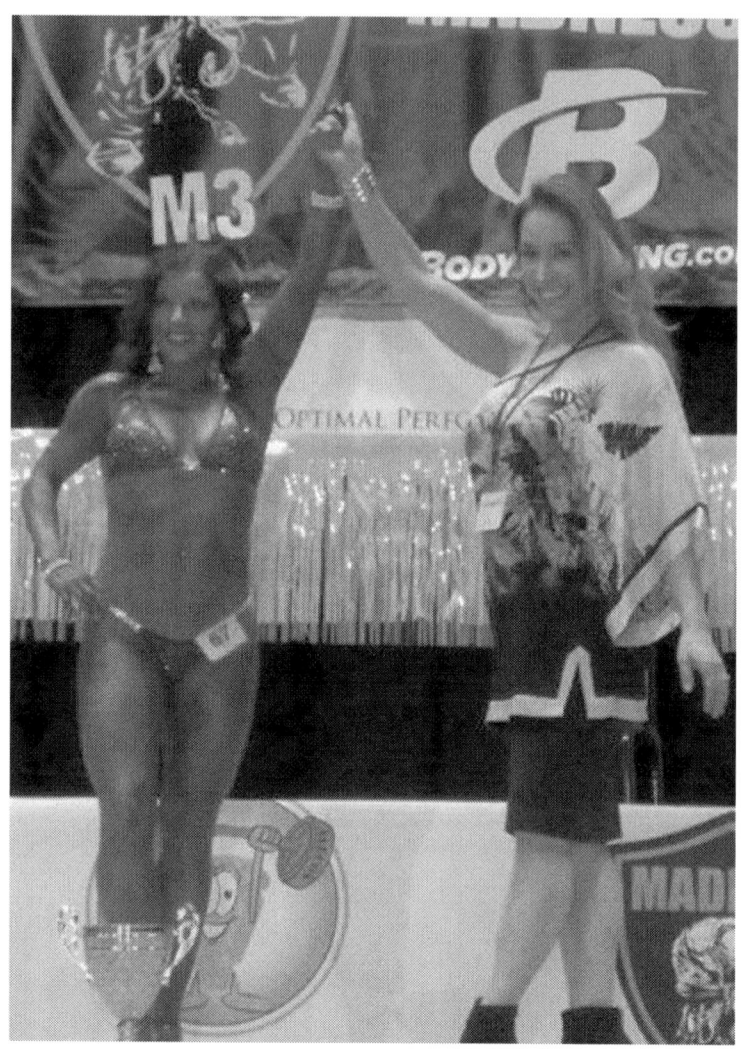

Other Exercise Models

We'd also like to thank Sophie Hurst and Rachel Bridge for volunteering to be our partner models to demonstrate the exercises with Helen Renée in this book.

Chapter 6: Exercise Resources
Stomach Muscles Partner Pole Pushdown

To perform the stomach muscles pole pushdown partners should stand upright facing each other, both with feet approximately shoulder-width apart and just over arm's length away from each other.

The supporting partner holds the pole horizontally typically with a palms-up handgrip and arms slightly bent, although this will vary according to the height of both partners. The partner performing the exercise should hold the middle of the pole with palms facing downwards, elbows slightly out and slightly bent in a locked position that will not change during the exercise.

In this position, the intention should be to press the pole down directly towards the ground. You do this by bending slightly at the waist to engage and use your stomach muscles to push the pole down. The harder you press and engage the stomach muscles, the more intense the exercise becomes, so be sure to exercise at an intensity that best suits you and your individual ability.

The harder you engage the muscles, the more intense the exercise becomes, so always be sure to exercise at an intensity that best suits your individual ability.

When you perform an isometric exercise never hold your breath. Always breathe deeply and naturally, which will be about 10 full breaths in and out at a rate of about 1 second per full breath. Perform each exercise for no less than 7 seconds, and for no longer than 10.

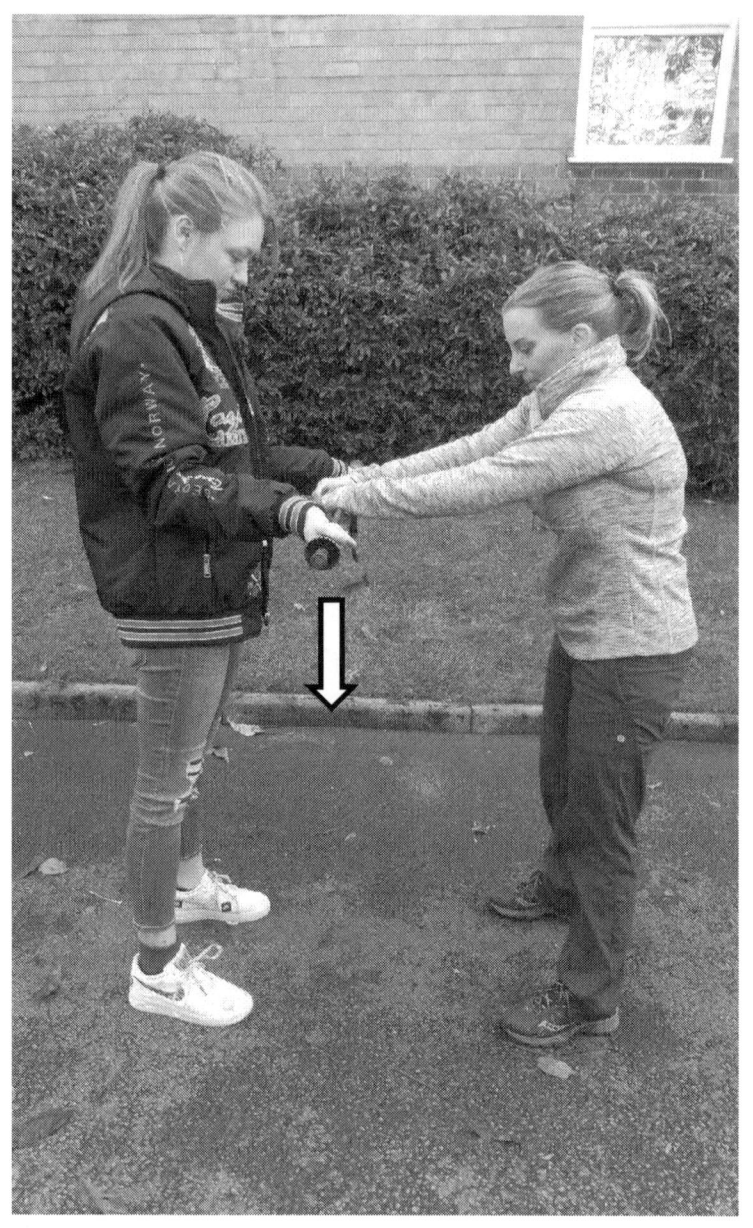

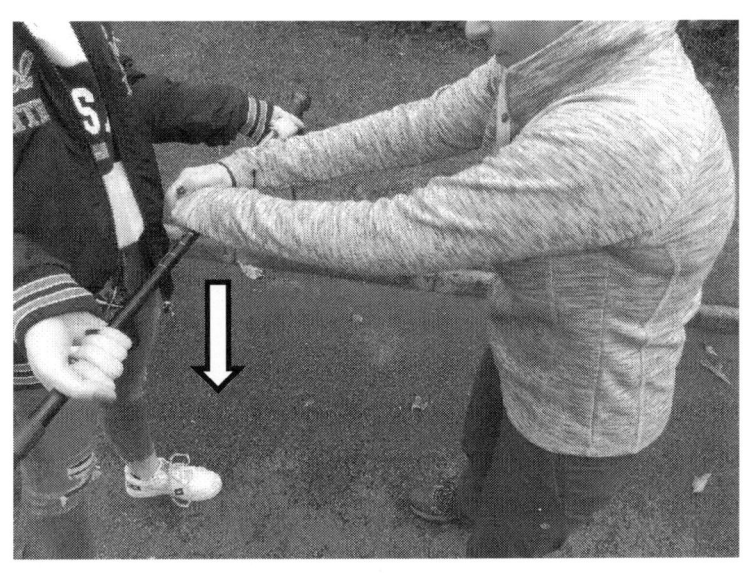

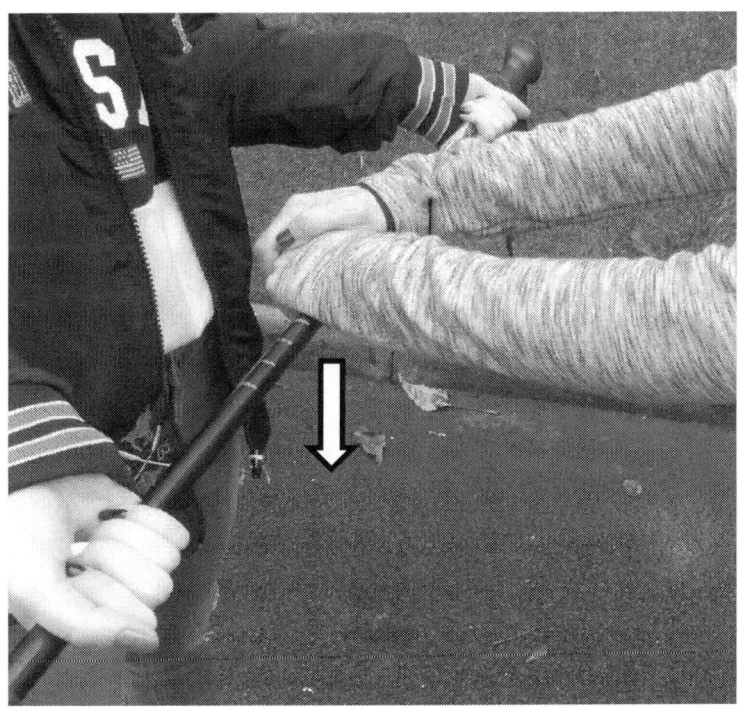

Arms – Upper Arm Partner Pole Under-Thigh Biceps Curl

To perform the partner upper arm pole under-thigh curl, both partners should stand upright touching each other back to back. One partner will act as a solid object to provide balance assistance to the other, therefore, they should form a foot brace position if possible to provide maximum stability.

The partner exercising should raise one leg in front of them with the knee bent. Slide the pole under that leg close to the bend in the knee. Hold the pole in both hands about shoulder-width apart with the palms facing up. In this position bend the arms in a curling motion until you reach the mid-point or maximum position you can attain. Even though you cannot raise the pole any further continue to try to do so and maintain a steady level of intensity to exercise the front upper arms. If necessary, you can always press downward with your bent raised leg to apply even more intensity to the arms during this exercise.

The harder you engage the muscles, the more intense the exercise becomes, so always be sure to exercise at an intensity that best suits your individual ability.

When you perform an isometric exercise never hold your breath. Always breathe deeply and naturally, which will be about 10 full breaths in and out at a rate of about 1 second per full breath. Perform each exercise for no less than 7 seconds, and for no longer than 10.

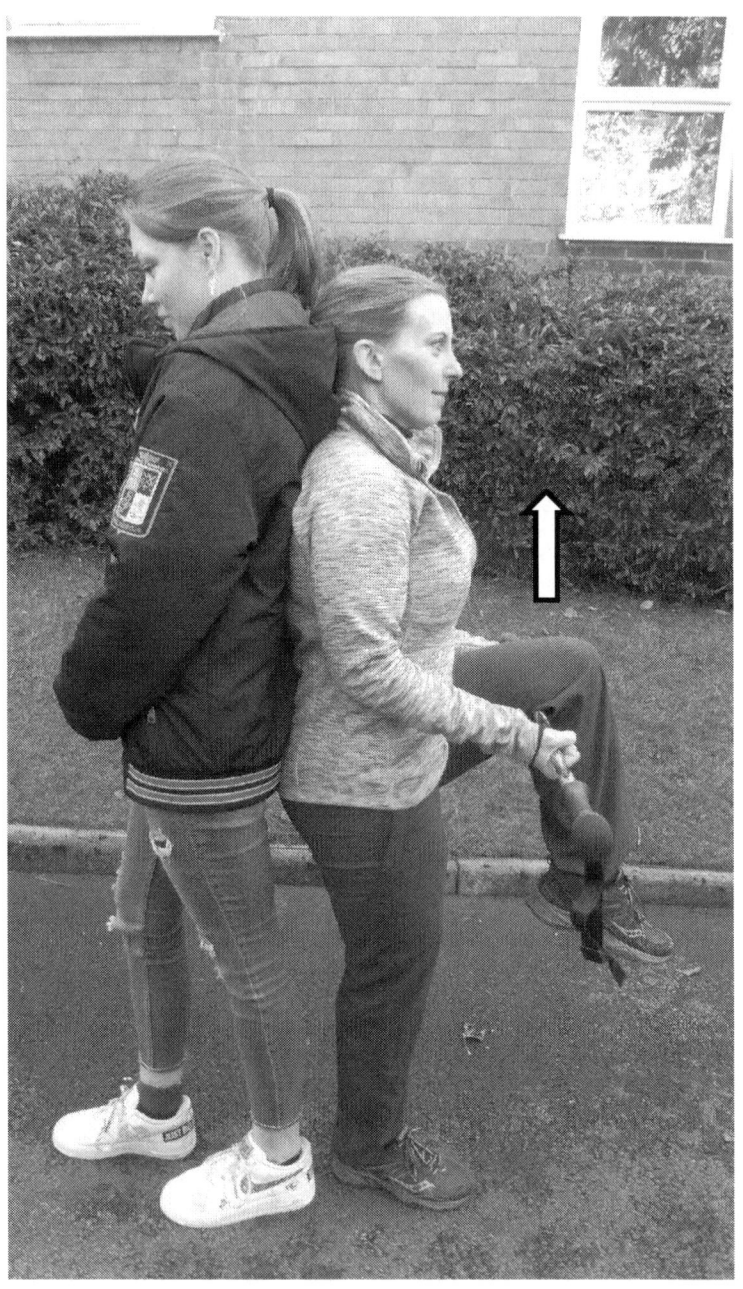

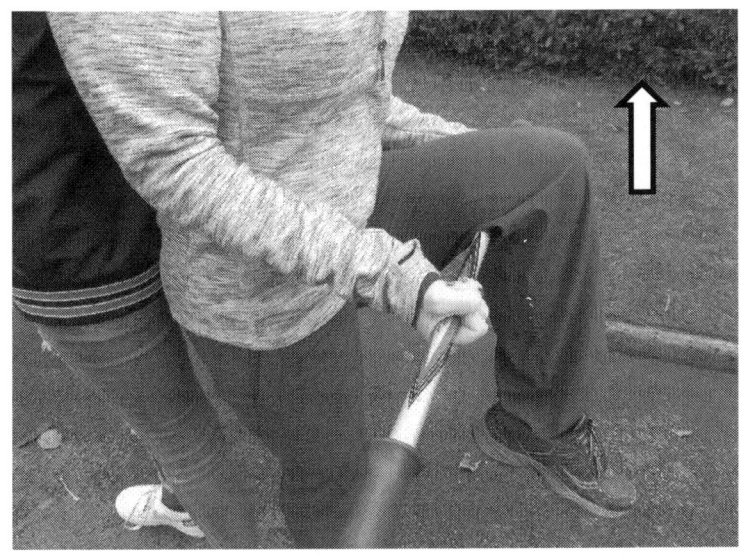

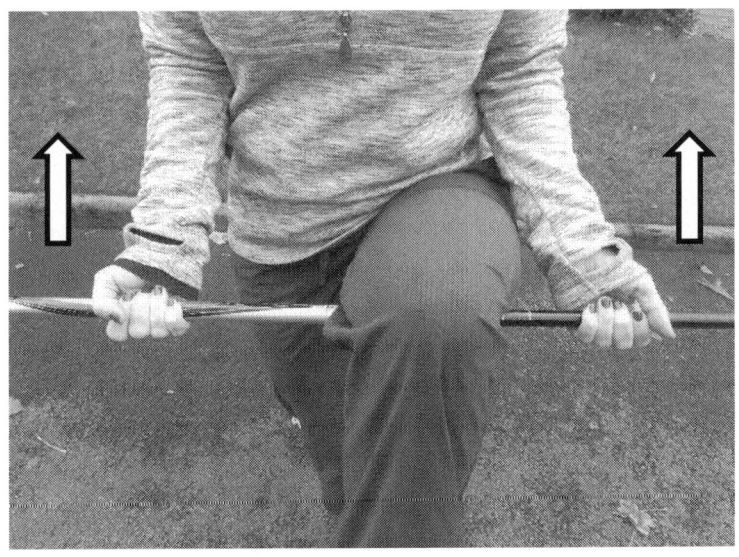

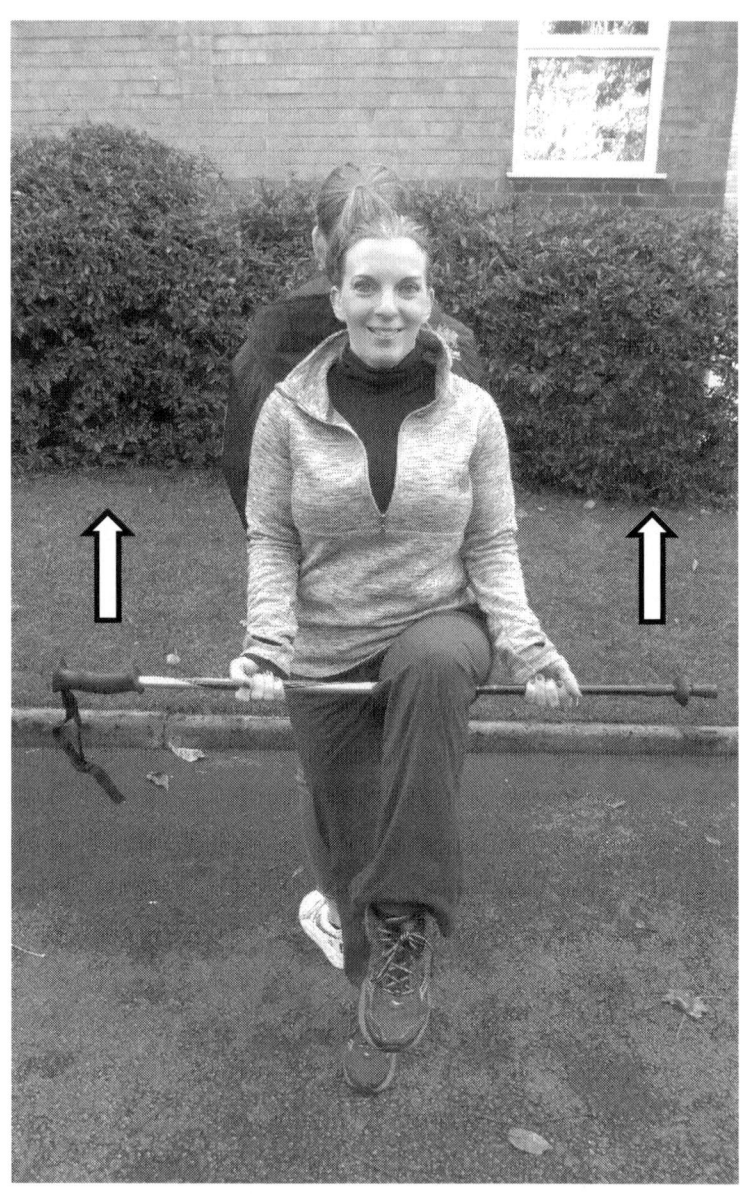

Arms
Upper Arm Partner Triceps-Biceps Curl-Press

The Upper arm triceps-biceps exercise engages both the front and rear upper arms. The exercise is in two parts. One part exercises the front upper arm of one side of the body and simultaneously the rear upper arm of the other side. In simple terms, one partner holds both of their hands at approximately mid-level with their elbows bent at approximately 90 degrees. One hand is facing upward, the other hand is facing downward. The other partner mirrors this position except that they have their hands in opposing directions so they can interlock hands. Exercise partners must stand face to face with each other so they can effectively interlock hands at the same height in order to perform the exercise. Be sure to always keep the arms roughly bent at midpoint with the elbows close to the body throughout the exercise. Always be sure that both partners exercise both arms/sides of the body equally in both directions. So, after a change of grip position and direction of effort, the emphasis of the exercise reverses for both partners.

The harder you press and engage both the biceps and triceps muscles, the more intense the exercise becomes, so be sure to grip firmly and exercise at an intensity that best suits your individual ability. When you perform an isometric exercise never hold your breath. Always breathe deeply and naturally, which will be about 10 full breaths in and out at a rate of about 1 second per full breath. Perform each exercise for no less than 7 seconds, and for no longer than 10.

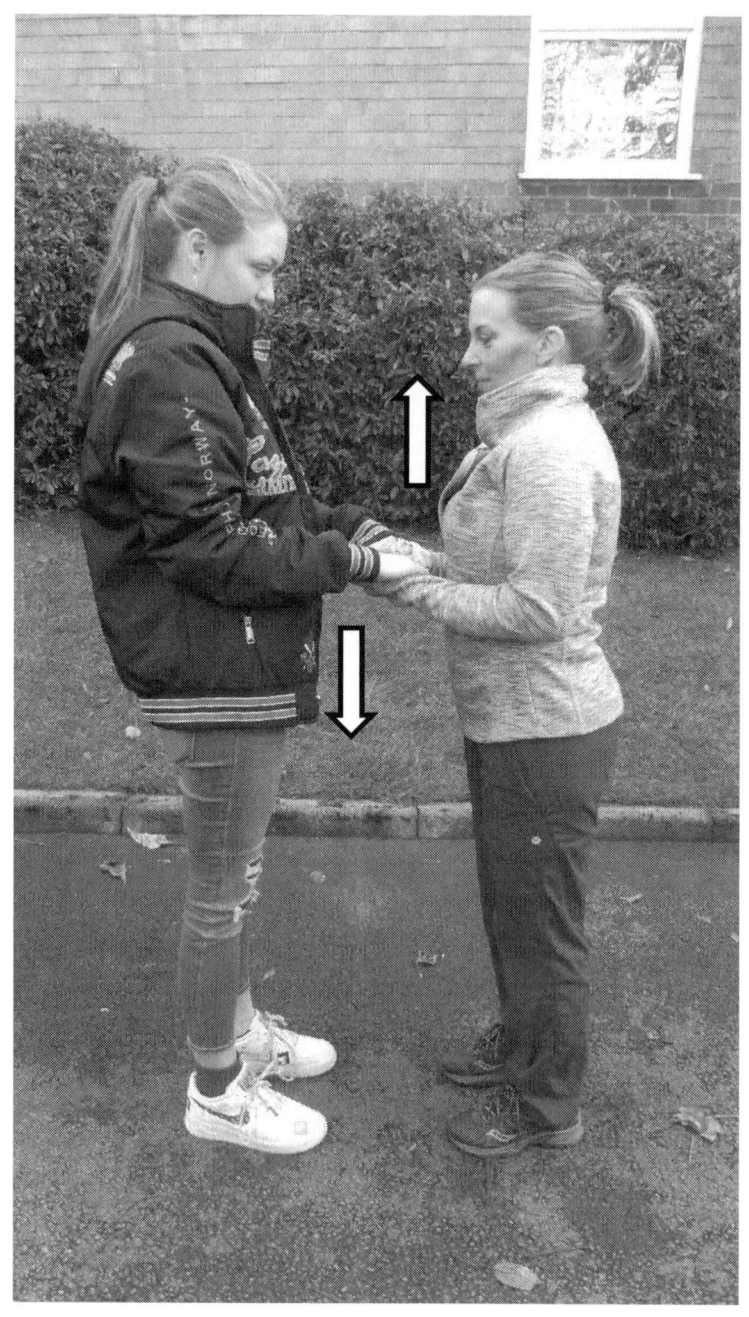

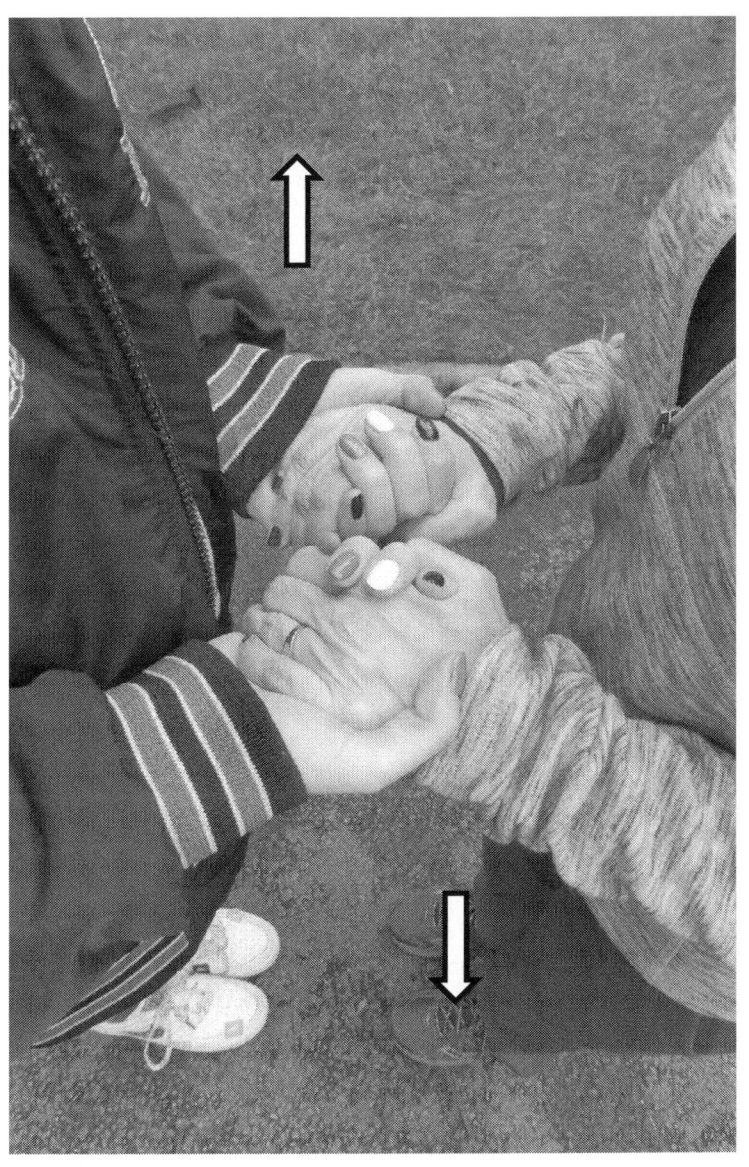

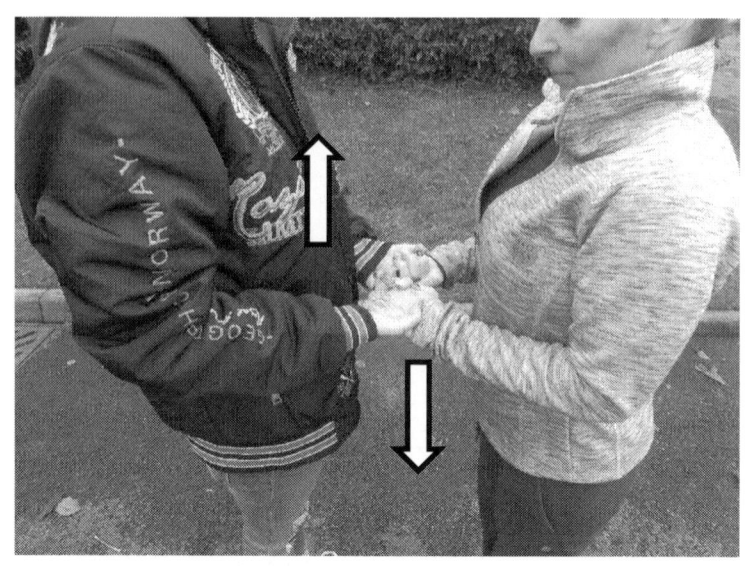

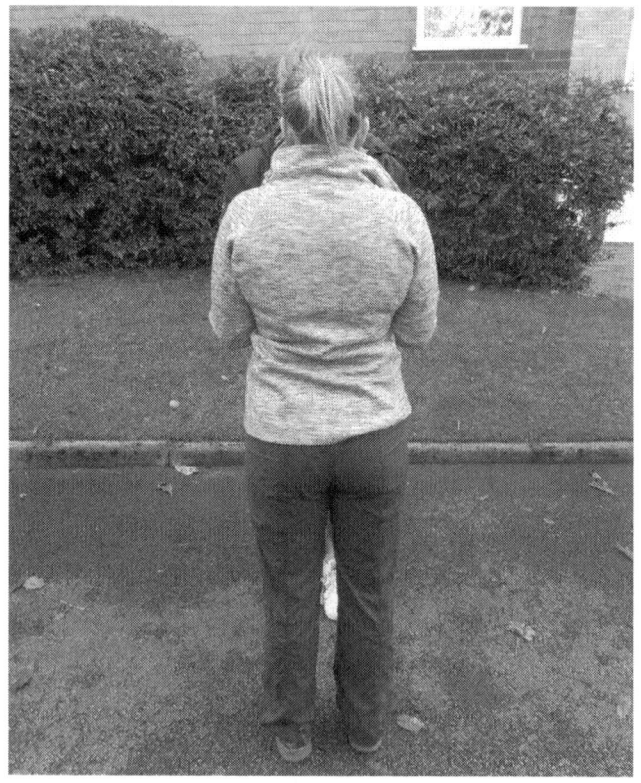

Arms
Upper Arm Partner Triceps-Biceps Pole Curl-Press

This exercise is essentially exactly the same as the previous exercise but instead of interlocking hands to perform the exercise, a pole is used instead. The Upper arm triceps-biceps exercise engages both the front and rear upper arms.

The exercise is in two parts. One part exercises the front upper arm of one side of the body and simultaneously the rear upper arm of the other side. In simple terms, one partner's arms/hands are attempting to raise up with their palms facing upward, and the other partner's arms/hands are pushing down with the palms facing down. Then, after a change of grip position and direction of effort, the emphasis of the exercise reverses.

Exercise partners must stand face to face with each other so they can effectively hold the pole at approximately the same height in order to perform the exercise. Always be sure that both partners exercise both arms/sides of the body equally in both directions. Be sure to always keep the arms roughly bent at midpoint with the elbows close to the body throughout the exercise.

The harder you engage the muscles, the more intense the exercise becomes, so always be sure to exercise at an intensity that best suits your individual ability. When you perform an isometric exercise never hold your breath. Always breathe deeply and naturally, which will be about 10 full breaths in and out at a rate of about 1 second per full breath. Perform each exercise for no less than 7 seconds, and for no longer than 10.

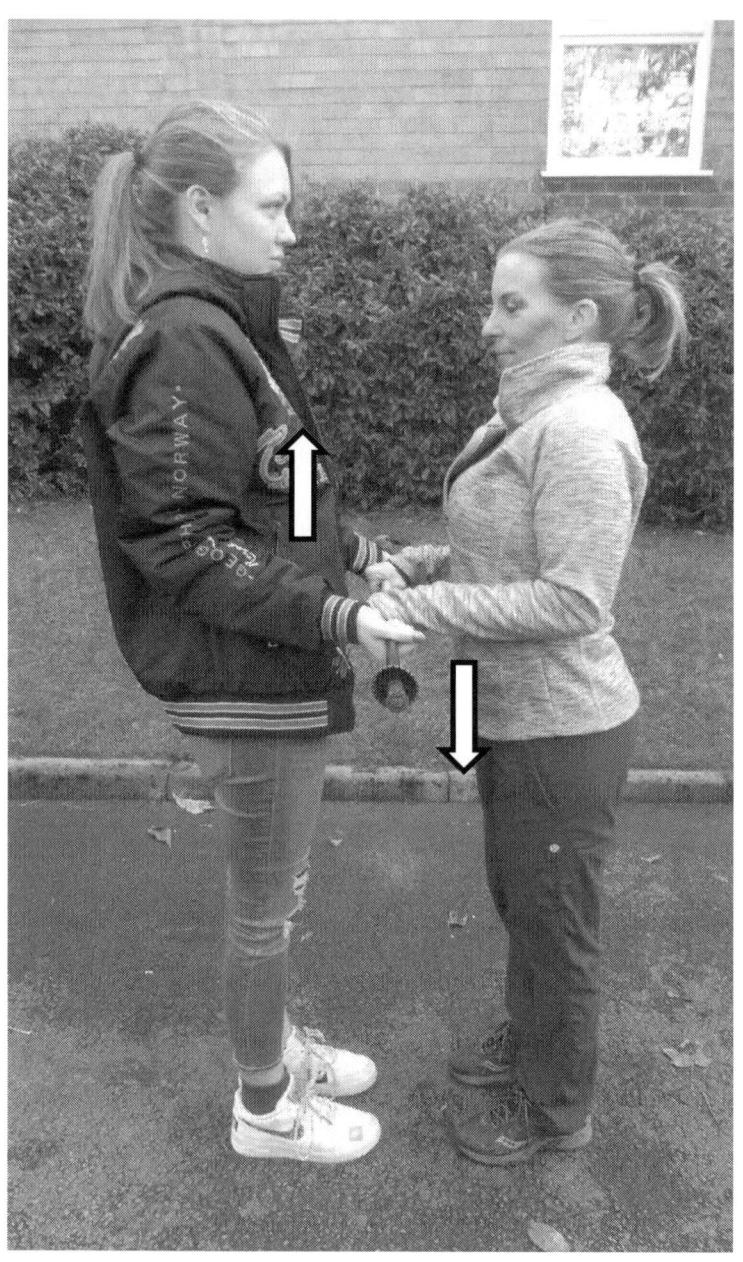

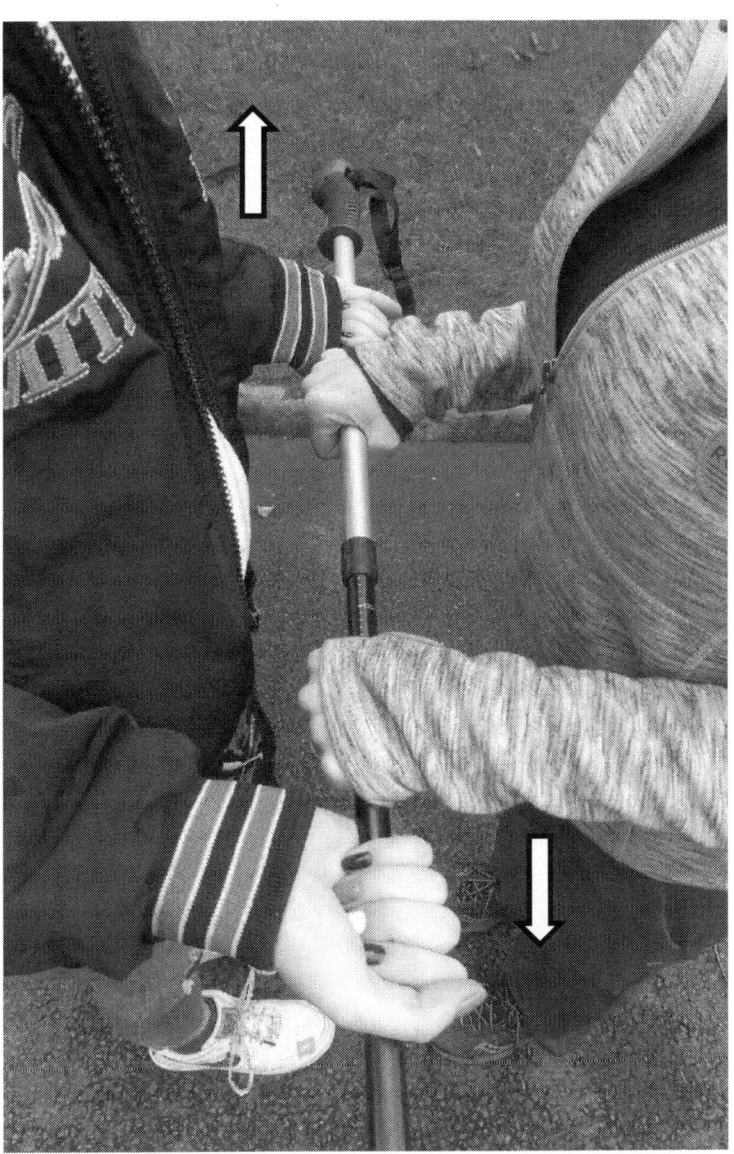

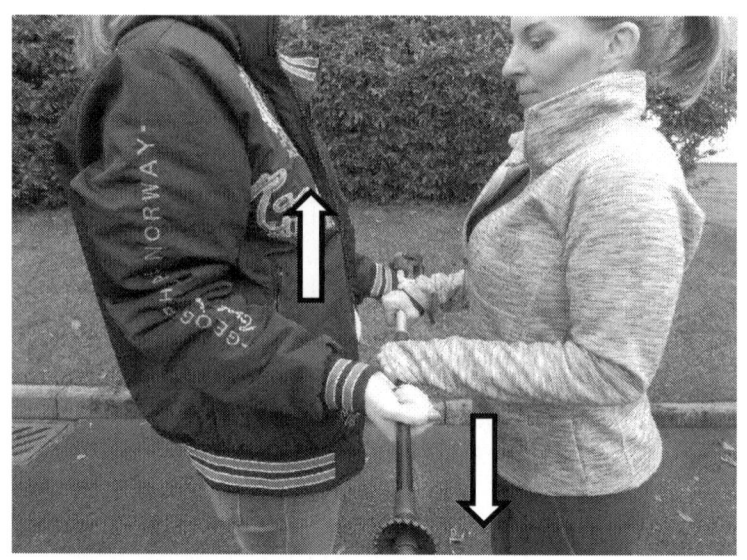

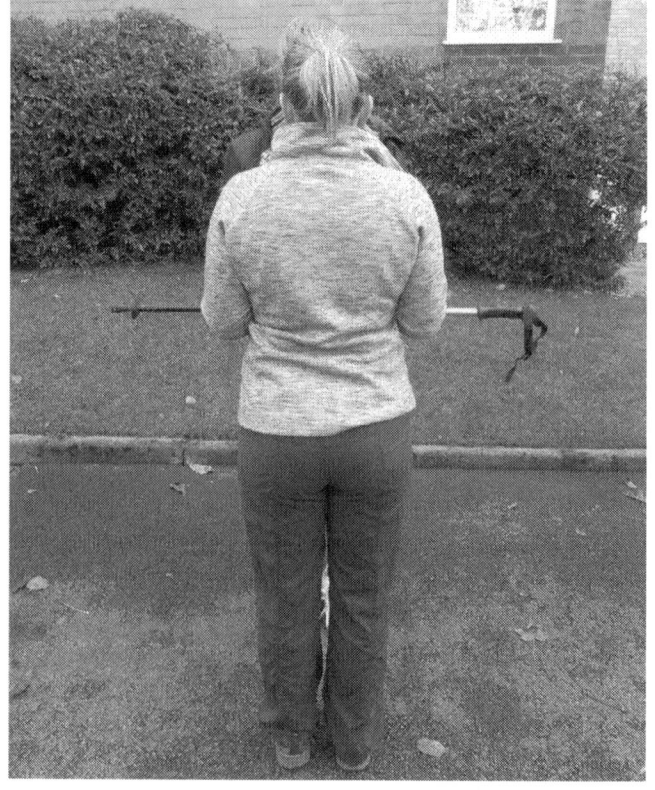

Arms
Upper Arm Triceps Partner-Pole Overhead Press

To perform this exercise the pole support partner must stand close behind the person performing the exercise. The partner performing the exercise should stand upright with the pole held vertically behind the back. The supporting partner holds the pole low behind the small of the exercising partners back. The exercising partner holds the pole over their overhead. The upper arms should be bent at approximately 90 degrees. In this position, the arms engage to try and press the pole upward with the overhead hands/arms engaging the triceps muscles to do this.

The harder you engage the muscles, the more intense the exercise becomes, so be sure to exercise at an intensity that best suits your individual ability. When you perform an isometric exercise never hold your breath. Always breathe deeply and naturally, which will be about 10 full breaths in and out at a rate of about 1 second per full breath. Perform each exercise for no less than 7 seconds, and for no longer than 10.

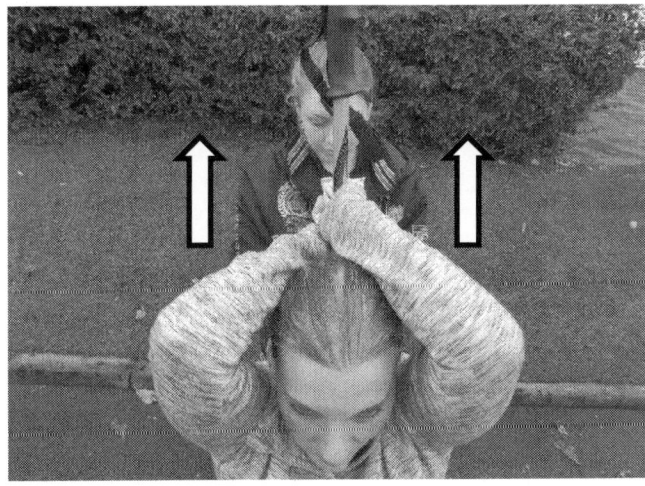

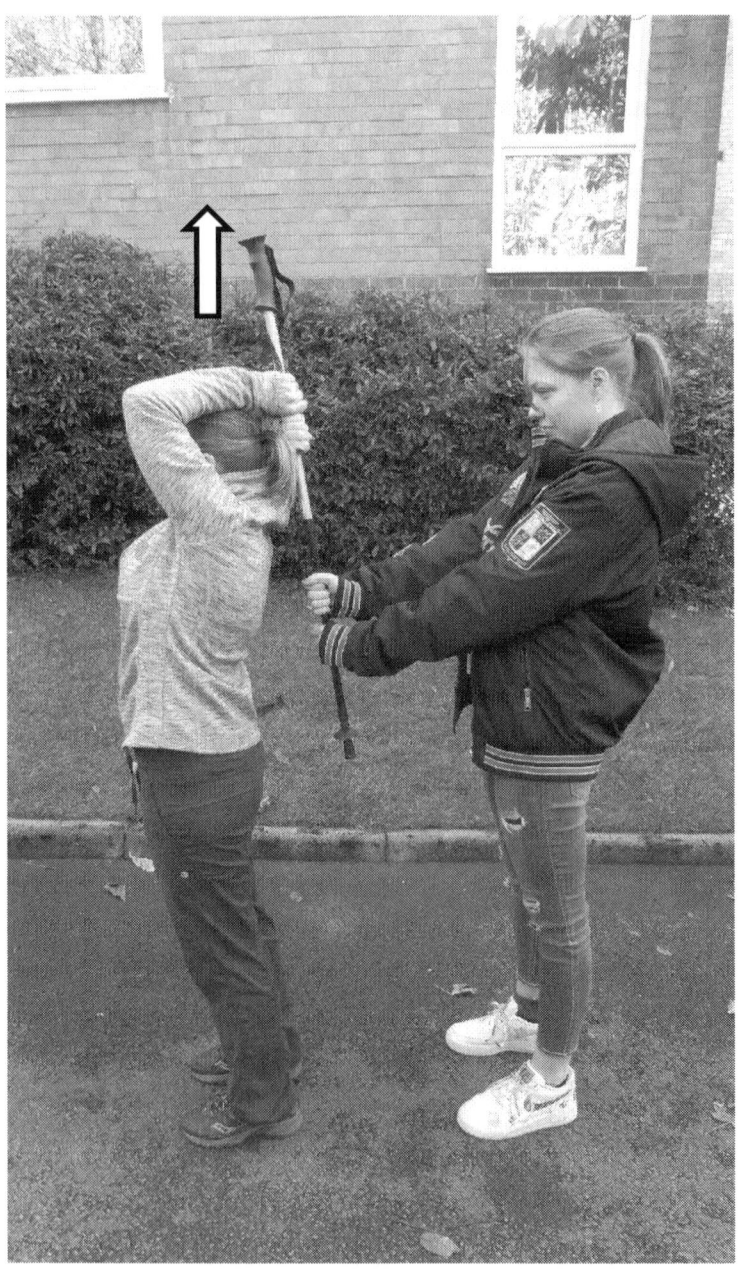

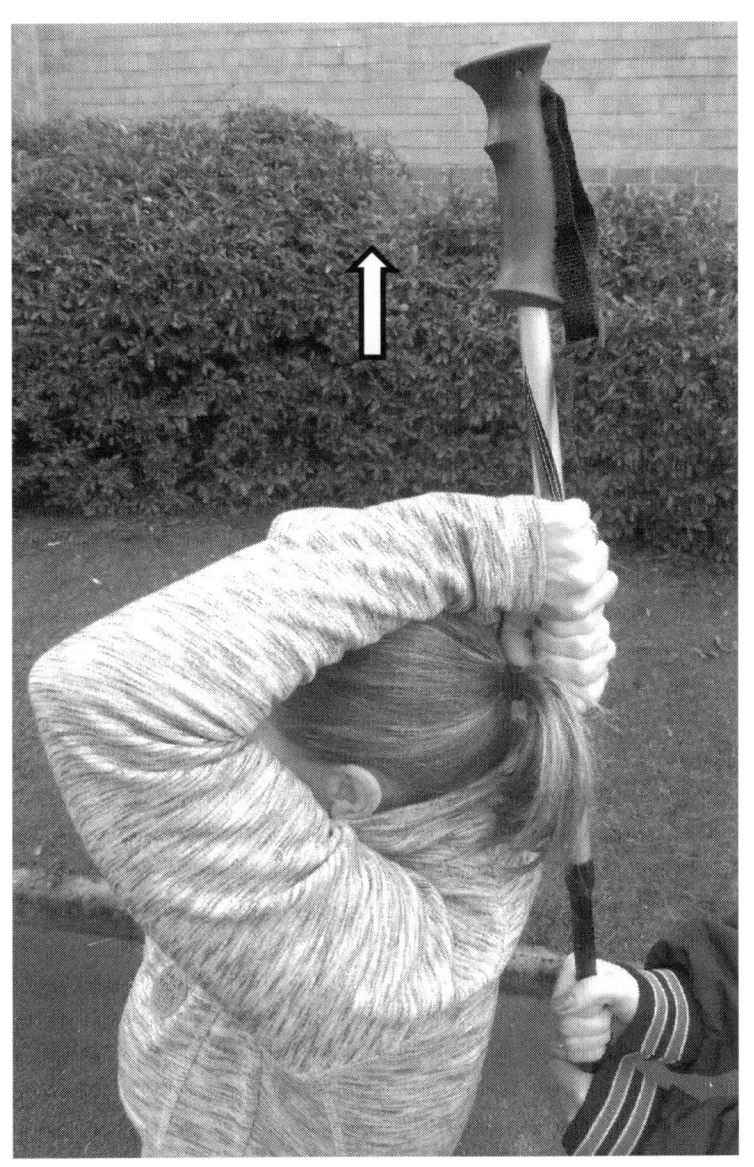

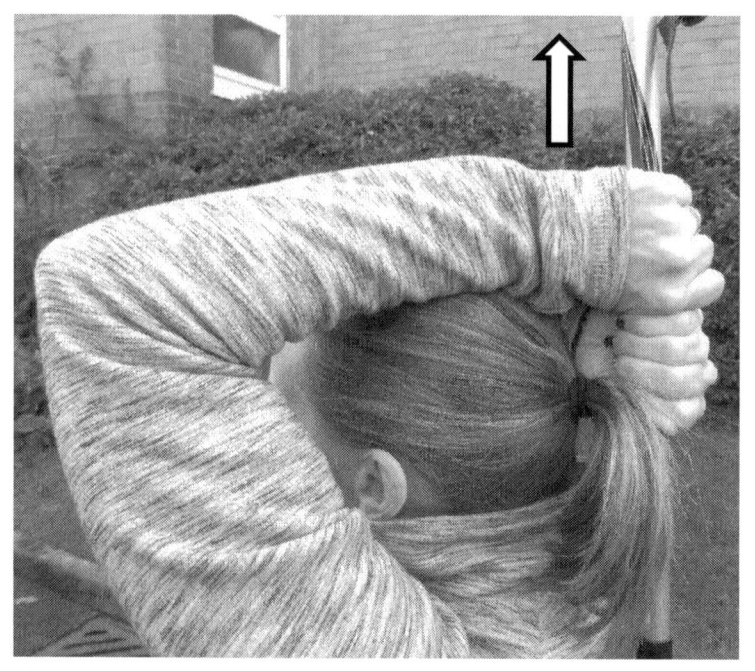

Lower Back
Partner Pole Good Morning Bend Over

     To perform this exercise both partners face each other sufficiently far apart that either party can bend over forwards without touching the other person. The exercising partner stands with their feet approximately shoulder-width apart and with their knees slightly bent. They bend forward only from the hip and always keep the back straight. The assisting partner places a pole evenly across the shoulders, never the neck, of the exercising partner. In that position, the exercising partner engages the lower back and buttock muscles as they gently attempt to raise back to the upright position. The assisting partner provides the agreed resistance so their partner can perform the exercise.

     The harder you engage the muscles, the more intense the exercise becomes, so always be sure to exercise at an intensity that best suits your individual ability. When you perform an isometric exercise never hold your breath. Always breathe deeply and naturally, which will be about 10 full breaths in and out at a rate of about 1 second per full breath. Perform each exercise for no less than 7 seconds, and for no longer than 10.

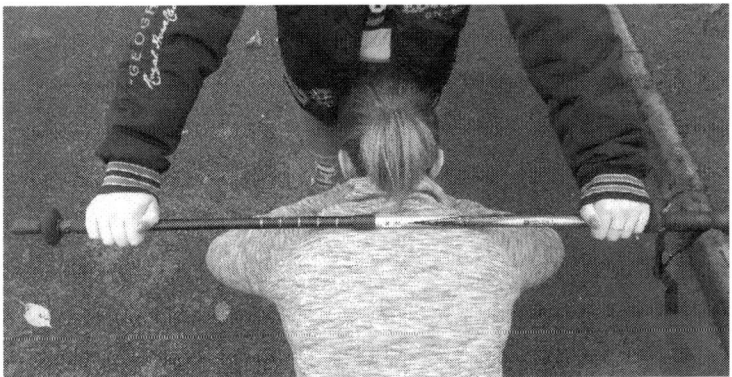

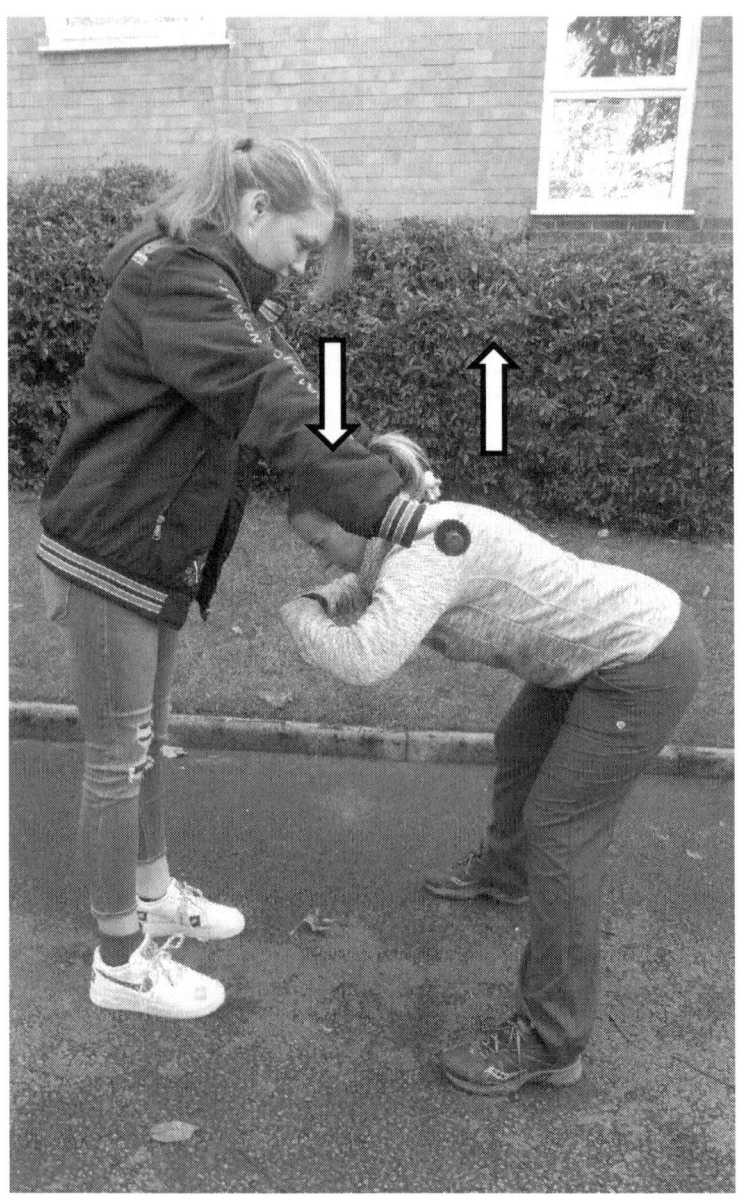

Upper Back
Partner Pole High-Level Pullback Row

To perform this exercise both partners face each other at approximate arm's length for both. Both the assisting partner and the exercising partner will technically both be exercising at the same time albeit in slightly different arm positions.

Both partners brace their stance with one foot slightly in front of the other to prevent them from being pulled forward during the exercise. Both partners hold the pole horizontally in front of them at approximately chest height, or a compromise height according to the height differential of the partners.

In this position, both partners pull the pole as if to pull it apart and at the same time pull the arms backwards in a rowing action. This will engage the upper back muscles. The final exercise position will typically be when one partner has their arms much more bent than the other, so they should always swap after each exercise so they both gain equal benefit from all positions.

The harder you engage the muscles, the more intense the exercise becomes, so always be sure to exercise at an intensity that best suits your individual ability.

When you perform an isometric exercise never hold your breath. Always breathe deeply and naturally, which will be about 10 full breaths in and out at a rate of about 1 second per full breath. Perform each exercise for no less than 7 seconds, and for no longer than 10.

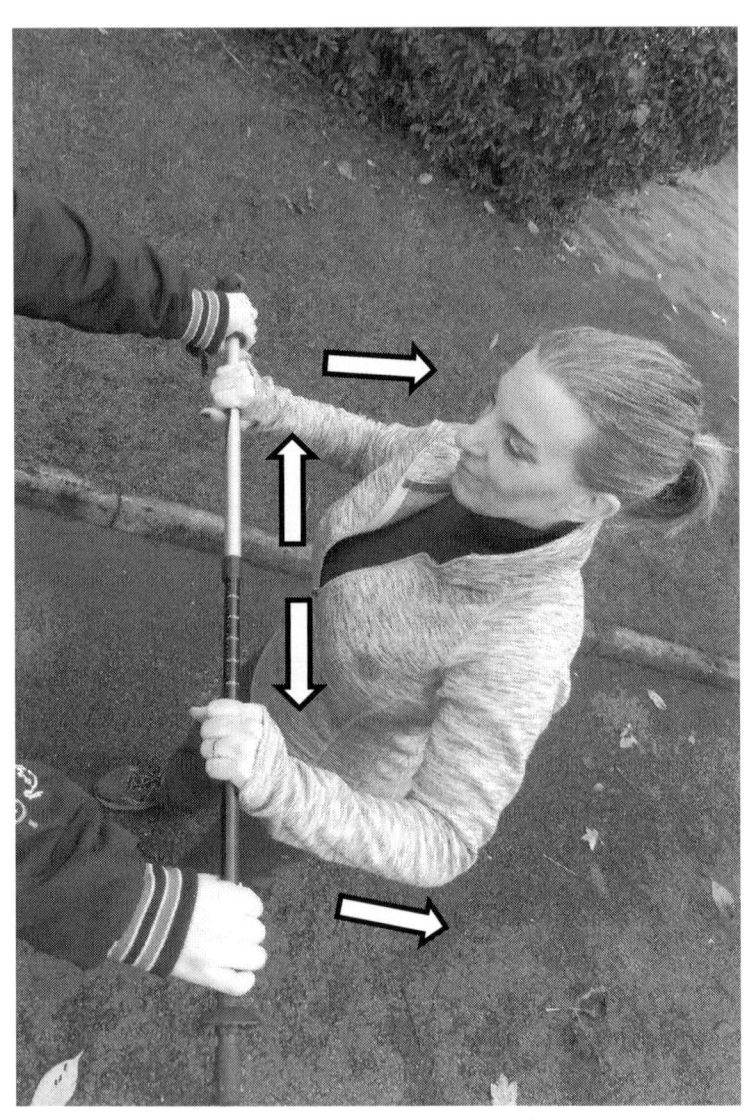

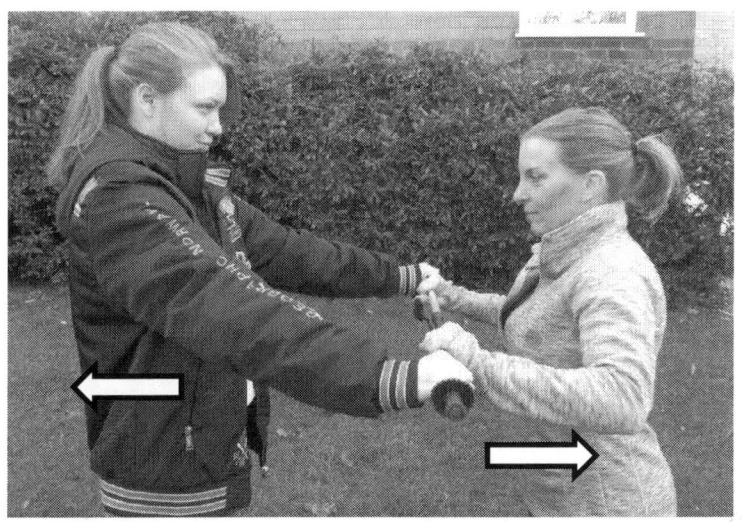

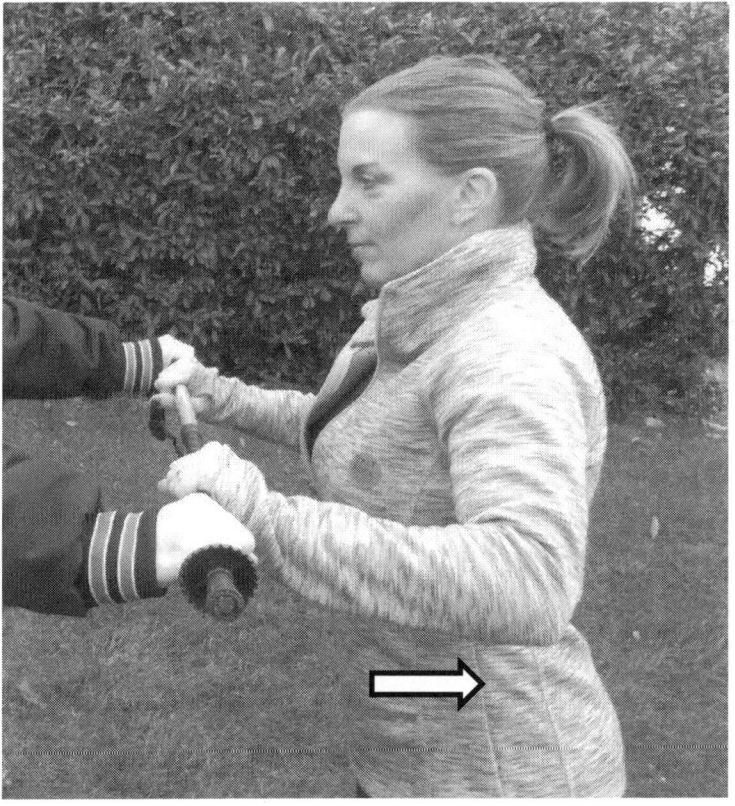

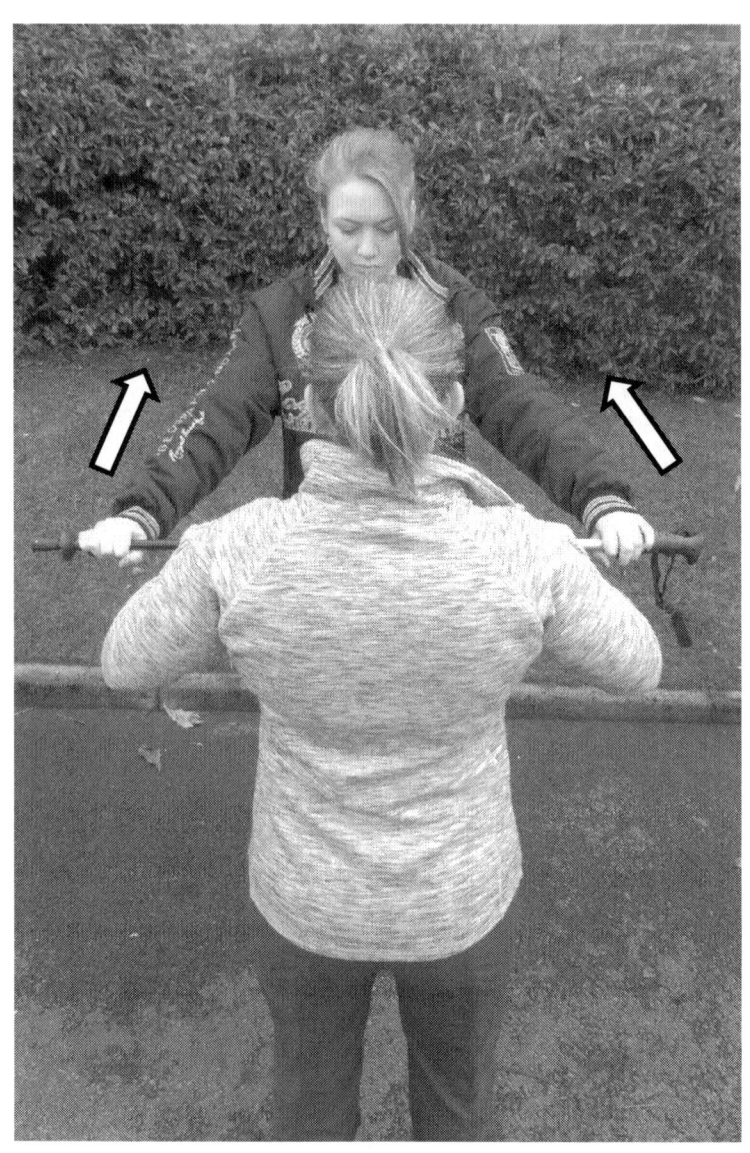

Chest - Partner Cross-Hand Chest Press

To perform this exercise both partners stand upright facing each other at a close distance. They both hold their arms and hands at chest height so their hands interlock. This means that the right hand of one partner interlocks palms with the right hand of the other partner, the left hands assume the same type of interlock. In this position, the forearms should be horizontal to the floor and the elbows raised to the side. Both partners press inwards with each resiting the other simultaneously pressing an interlocked palm against palm. This will engage the chest muscles.

The harder you engage the muscles, the more intense the exercise becomes, so always be sure to exercise at an intensity that best suits your individual ability. When you perform an isometric exercise never hold your breath. Always breathe deeply and naturally, which will be about 10 full breaths in and out at a rate of about 1 second per full breath. Perform each exercise for no less than 7 seconds, and for no longer than 10.

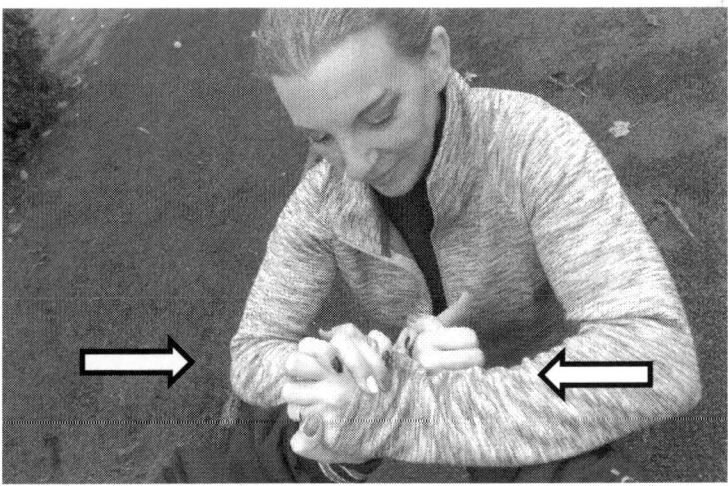

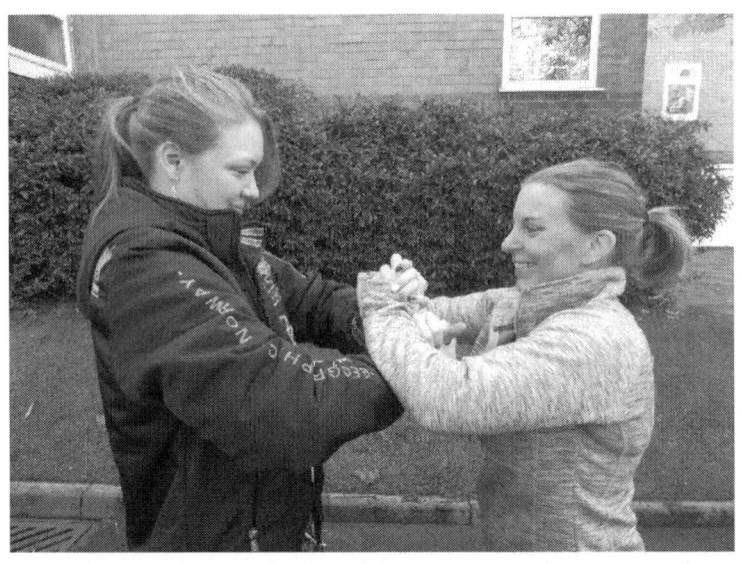

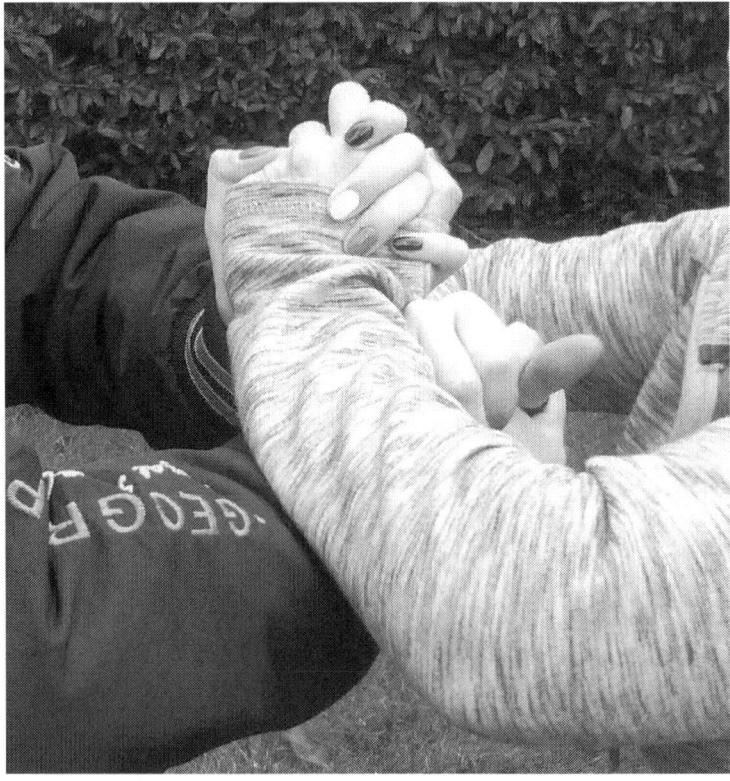

Chest - Partner Pole Chest Press

To perform this exercise both partners face each other at approximate arm's length for both. Both the assisting partner and the exercising partner will technically both be exercising at the same time albeit in slightly different arm positions.

Both partners brace their stance with one foot slightly in front of the other to prevent them from being pushed back during the exercise. Both partners hold the pole horizontally in front of them at approximately chest height, or a compromise height according to the height differential of the partners. Both partners grip the pole wider than shoulder-width apart so that when their arms are bent at mid-point they assume a 90-degree angle.

In this position, both partners push each other with equal force as if performing a push-up action. This will engage the chest muscles. Both partners must agree when to disengage from the exercise to prevent the other from suddenly falling face-forwards to the floor if one party stops the exercise abruptly for any reason. This is also another good reason why both partners should brace their stance with one foot/leg slightly in front of the other.

The harder you engage the muscles, the more intense the exercise becomes, so always be sure to exercise at an intensity that best suits your individual ability.

When you perform an isometric exercise never hold your breath. Always breathe deeply and naturally, which will be about 10 full breaths in and out at a rate of about 1 second per full breath. Perform each exercise for no less than 7 seconds, and for no longer than 10.

98

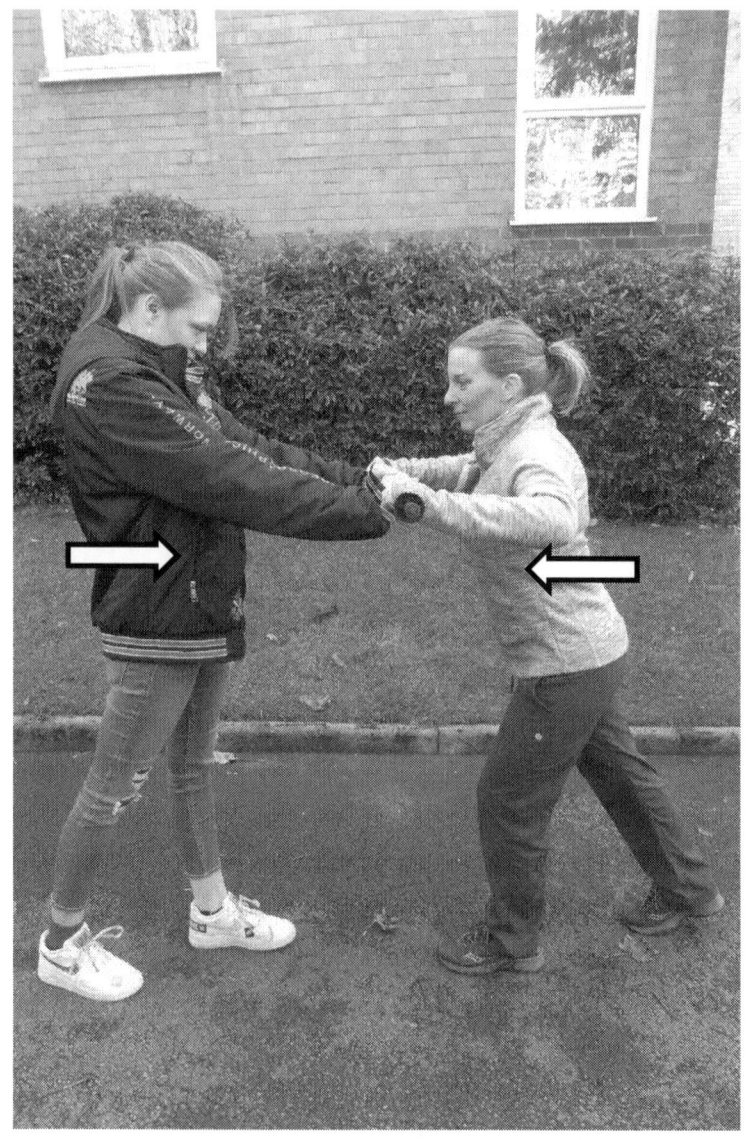

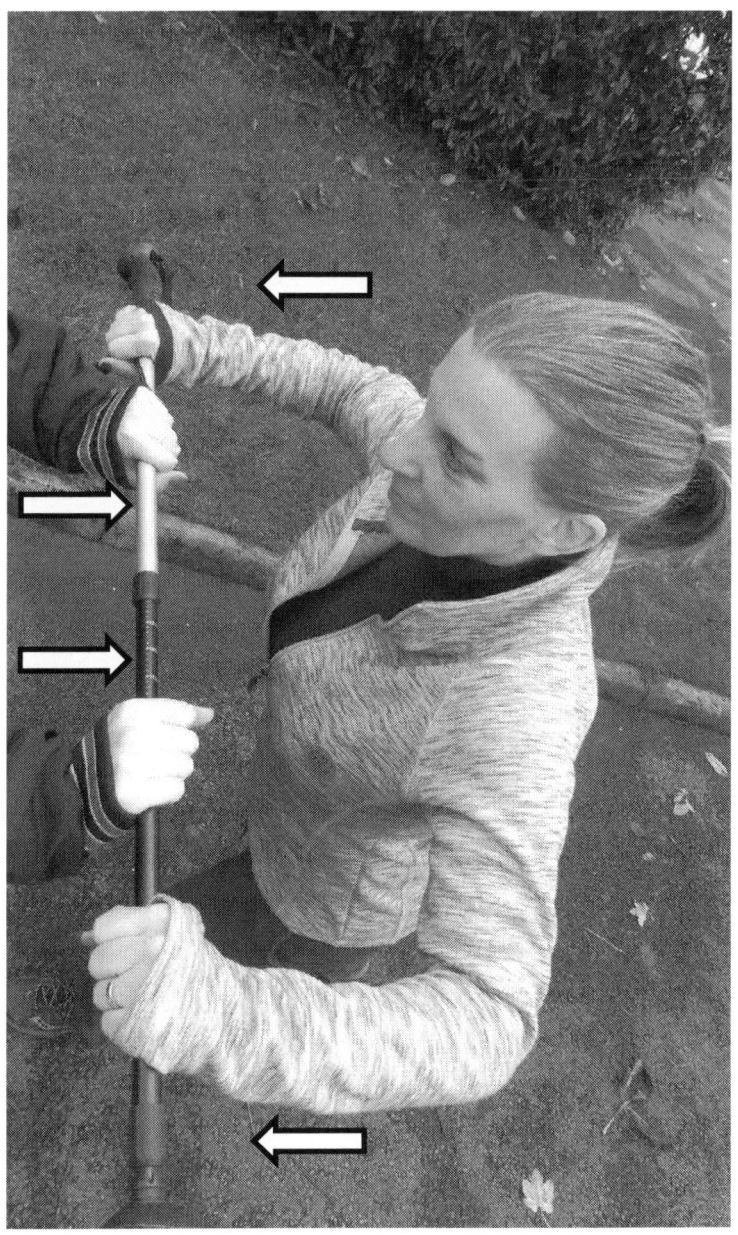

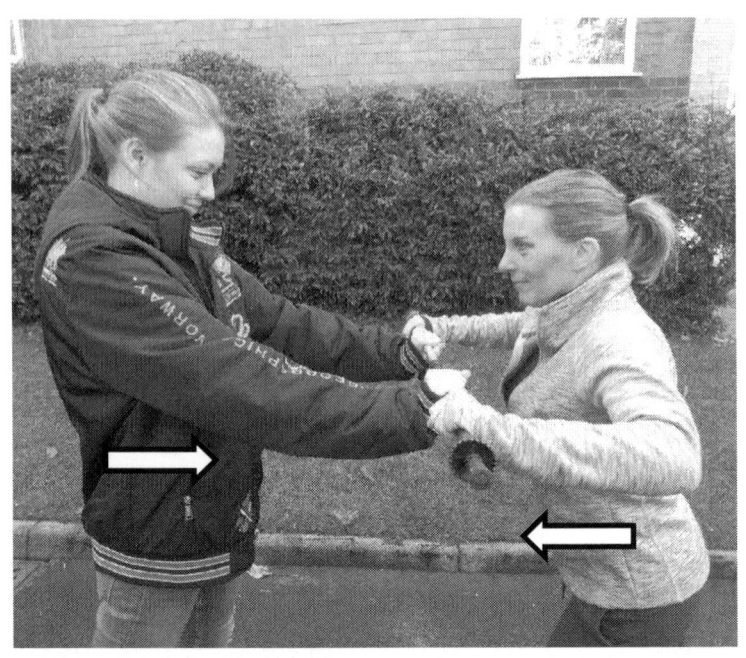

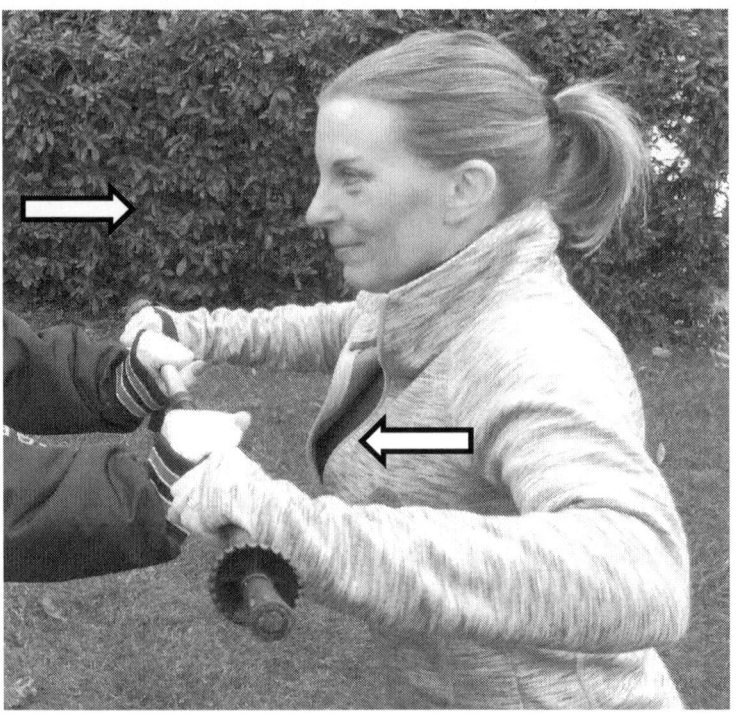

Legs – Calf Muscles
Partner Pole Double Heel Raise

To perform this exercise both partners face each other at approximate arm's length for both. Both the assisting partner and the exercising partner can if they wish technically both be exercising at the same time albeit in slightly different arm positions. However, it's not recommended unless both partners have excellent balance. Typically, the supporting partner will use the horizontally held pole as an object for the exercising partner to use as a focussed balance aid. The exercising partner will stand with feet approximately shoulder-width apart. They will then perform a double heel raise onto the balls of both feet. If the supporting partner is braced to resist a push, then the exercising partner may also use the calf muscle to press forward slightly at the same time.

In this position, both partners support or counter push each other with equal force. Both partners must agree when to disengage from the exercise to prevent the other from suddenly falling face-forwards to the floor if one party stops the exercise abruptly for any reason. This is also another good reason why both partners should brace their stance with one foot/leg slightly in front of the other. The harder you engage the muscles, the more intense the exercise becomes, so always be sure to exercise at an intensity that best suits your individual ability. When you perform an isometric exercise never hold your breath. Always breathe deeply and naturally, which will be about 10 full breaths in and out at a rate of about 1 second per full breath. Perform each exercise for no less than 7 seconds, and for no longer than 10.

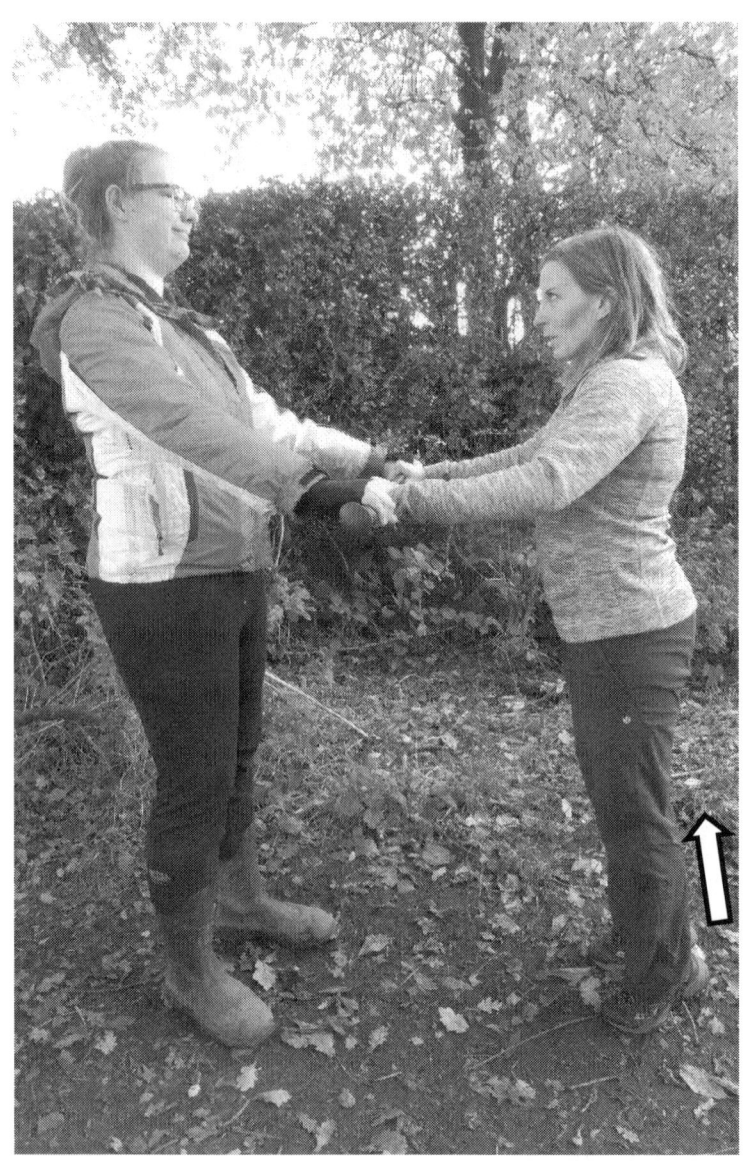

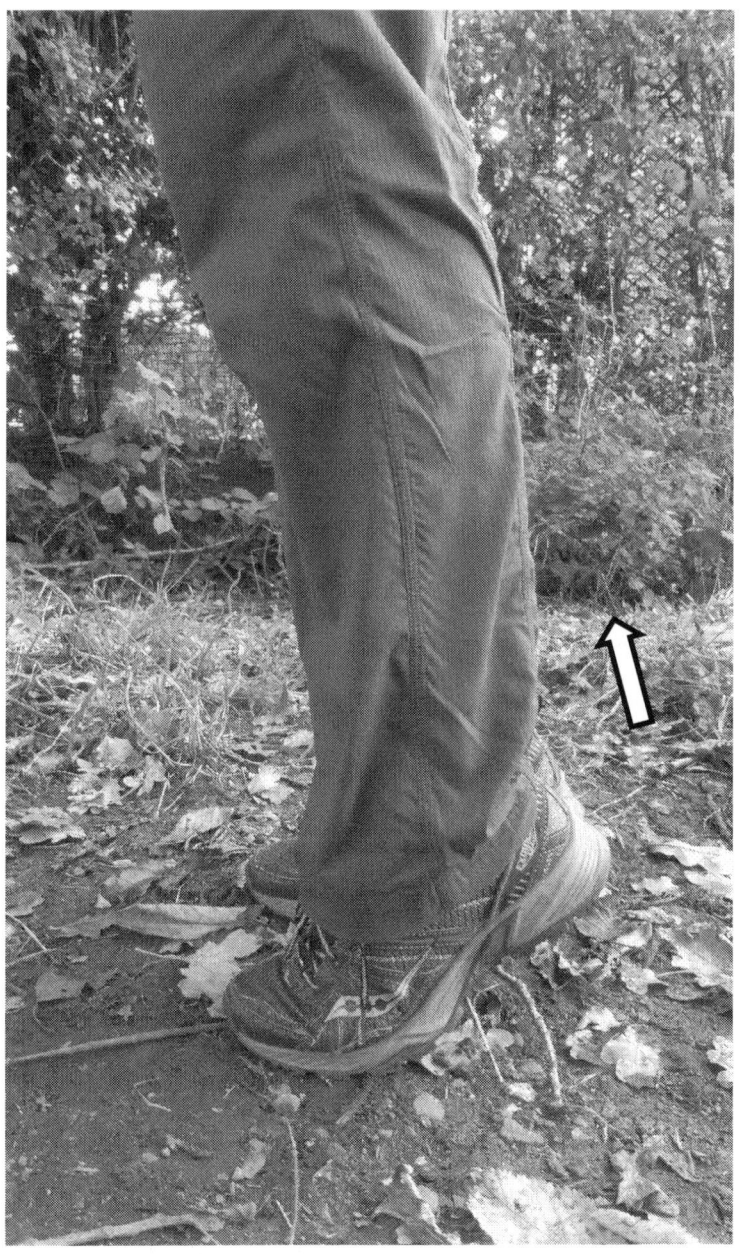

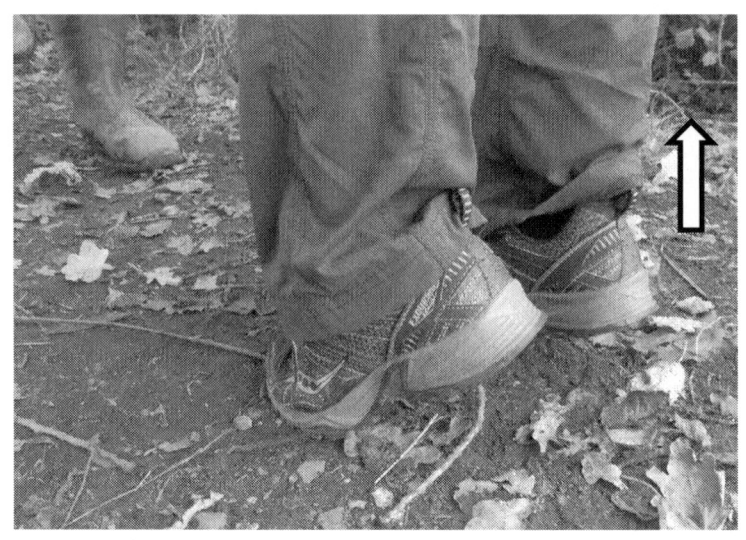

Legs – Calf Muscles
Partner Pole Single Heel Raise

To perform this exercise both partners face each other at approximate arm's length for both. Both the assisting partner and the exercising partner can if they wish technically both be exercising at the same time albeit in slightly different arm positions. However, it's not recommended unless both partners have excellent balance. Typically, the supporting partner will use the horizontally held pole as an object for the exercising partner to use as a focussed balance aid. The exercising partner will stand with feet approximately shoulder-width apart. They will then perform a single heel raise onto the ball of one foot. If the supporting partner is braced to resist a push, then the exercising partner may also use the calf muscle to press forward slightly at the same time.

In this position, both partners support or counter push each other with equal force. Both partners must agree when to disengage from the exercise to prevent the other from suddenly falling face-forwards to the floor if one party stops the exercise abruptly for any reason. This is also another good reason why both partners should brace their stance with one foot/leg slightly in front of the other. The harder you engage the muscles, the more intense the exercise becomes, so always be sure to exercise at an intensity that best suits your individual ability. When you perform an isometric exercise never hold your breath. Always breathe deeply and naturally, which will be about 10 full breaths in and out at a rate of about 1 second per full breath. Perform each exercise for no less than 7 seconds, and for no longer than 10.

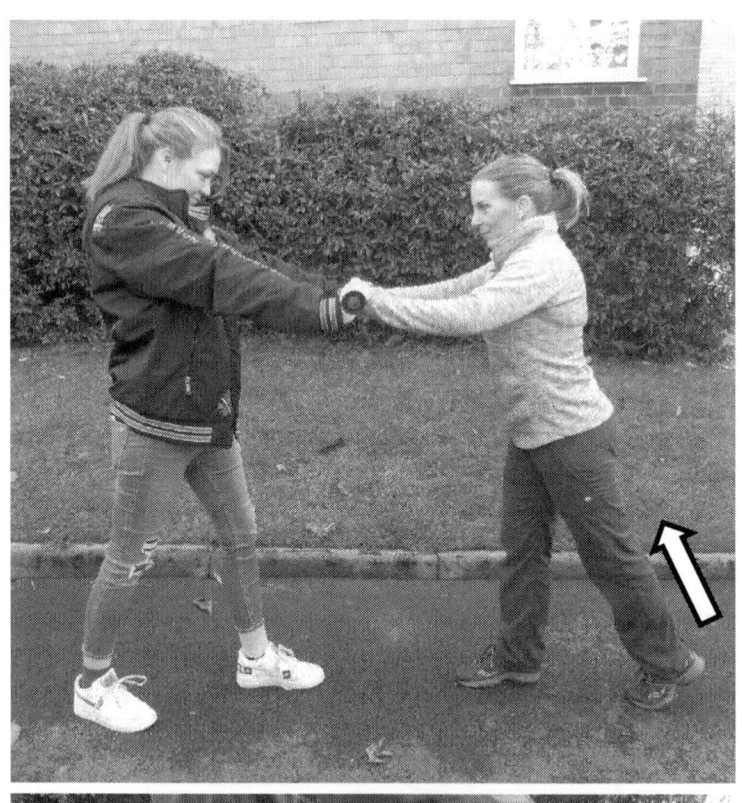

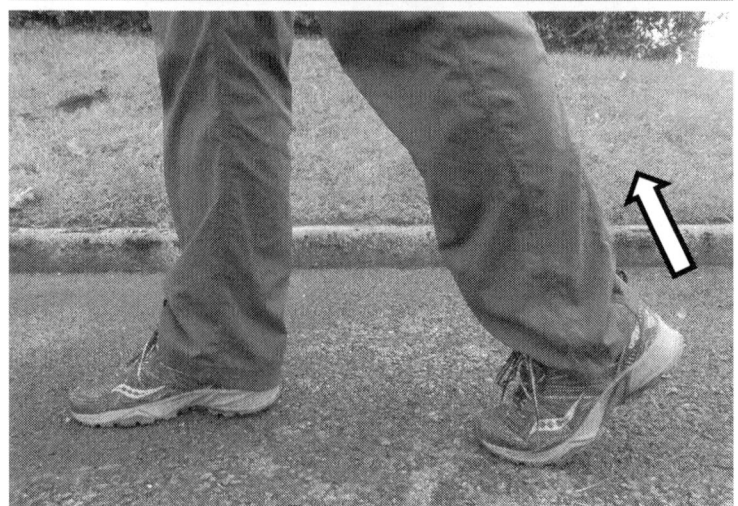

Legs – Thighs - Partner Pole Lunge

To perform this exercise both partners face each other at approximate arm's length for both. The pole is held horizontally at a mutually agreed height according to the height differential of both partners.

The exercising partner stands with their feet approximately shoulder-width apart. They hold the pole lightly to assist with balance and only if needed. They step straight forward with one leg bending into a lunge position that is as deep as can comfortably and safely be achieved.

Hold the bent-knee lunge position to exercise the front upper thigh and the buttocks. Be sure to exercise both sides of the body.

Both partners must agree when to disengage from the exercise to prevent the other from suddenly losing balance and possibly even falling if one party stops the exercise abruptly for any reason.

The harder you engage the muscles, the more intense the exercise becomes, so always be sure to exercise at an intensity that best suits your individual ability.

When you perform an isometric exercise never hold your breath. Always breathe deeply and naturally, which will be about 10 full breaths in and out at a rate of about 1 second per full breath. Perform each exercise for no less than 7 seconds, and for no longer than 10.

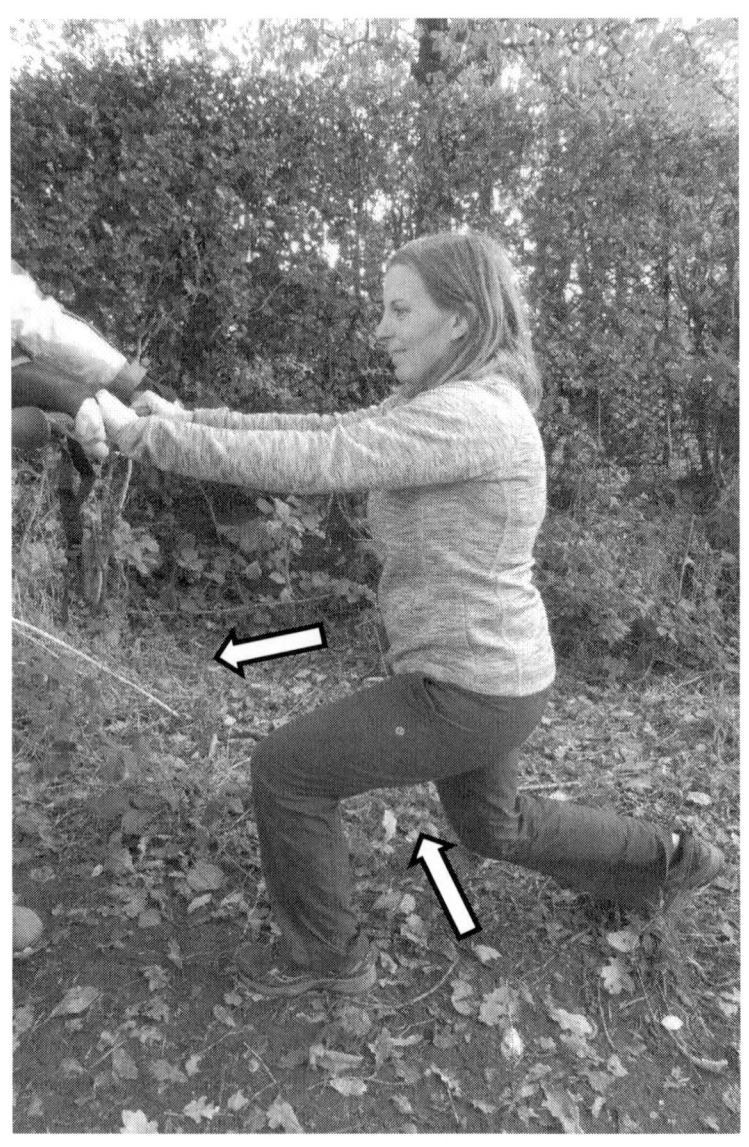

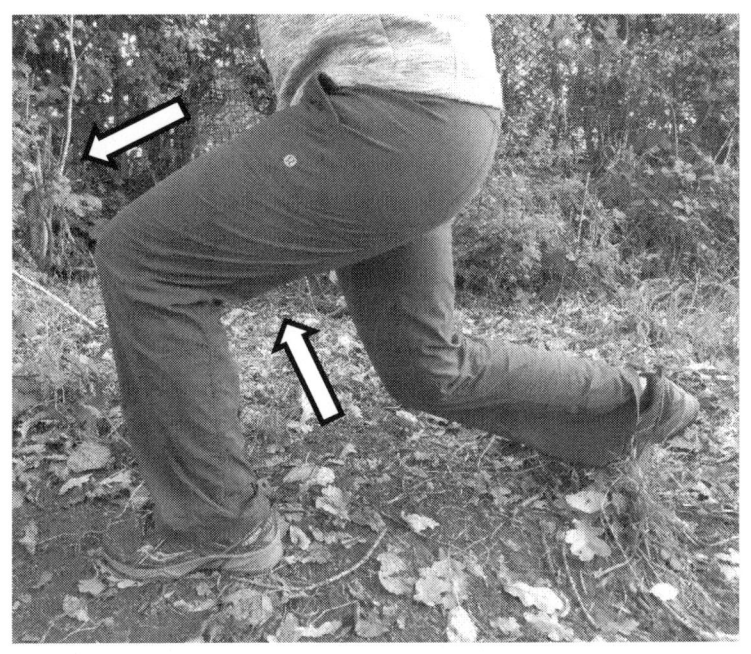

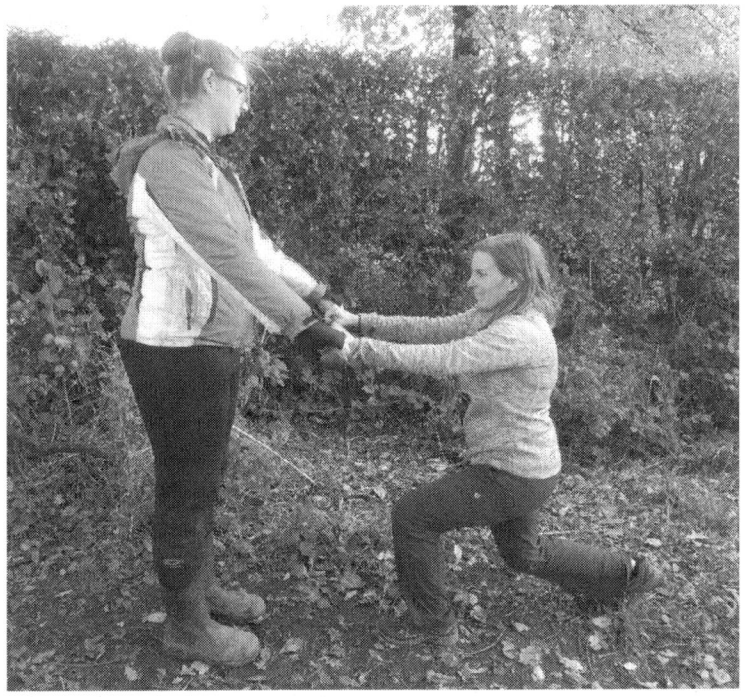

Legs – Thighs - Partner Pole Assisted Squat

To perform this exercise both partners face each other at approximate arm's length for both. The pole is held horizontally at a mutually agreed height according to the height differential of both partners. The exercising partner stands with their feet approximately shoulder-width apart. They hold the pole lightly to assist with balance and if needed, to assist if they need help holding a squat position. The exercising partner bends the knees and assumes a squat position, ideally with the thighs parallel to the floor or as near to that as possible. As they squat they keep their back straight and bend forward only from the hips. The squat position is then held to perform the exercise.

Some people may either intentionally or inadvertently lean backward as they squat due to flexibility issues in their knees, ankles and hips. For this reason, the assisting partner must be aware of this possibility and brace their stance to accommodate for any shift in weight that may follow if their exercising partner does this. Both partners must agree when to disengage from the exercise to prevent the other from suddenly losing balance and possibly even falling if one party stops the exercise abruptly for any reason. The harder you engage the muscles, the more intense the exercise becomes, so always be sure to exercise at an intensity that best suits your individual ability. When you perform an isometric exercise never hold your breath. Always breathe deeply and naturally, which will be about 10 full breaths in and out at a rate of about 1 second per full breath. Perform each exercise for no less than 7 seconds, and for no longer than 10.

112

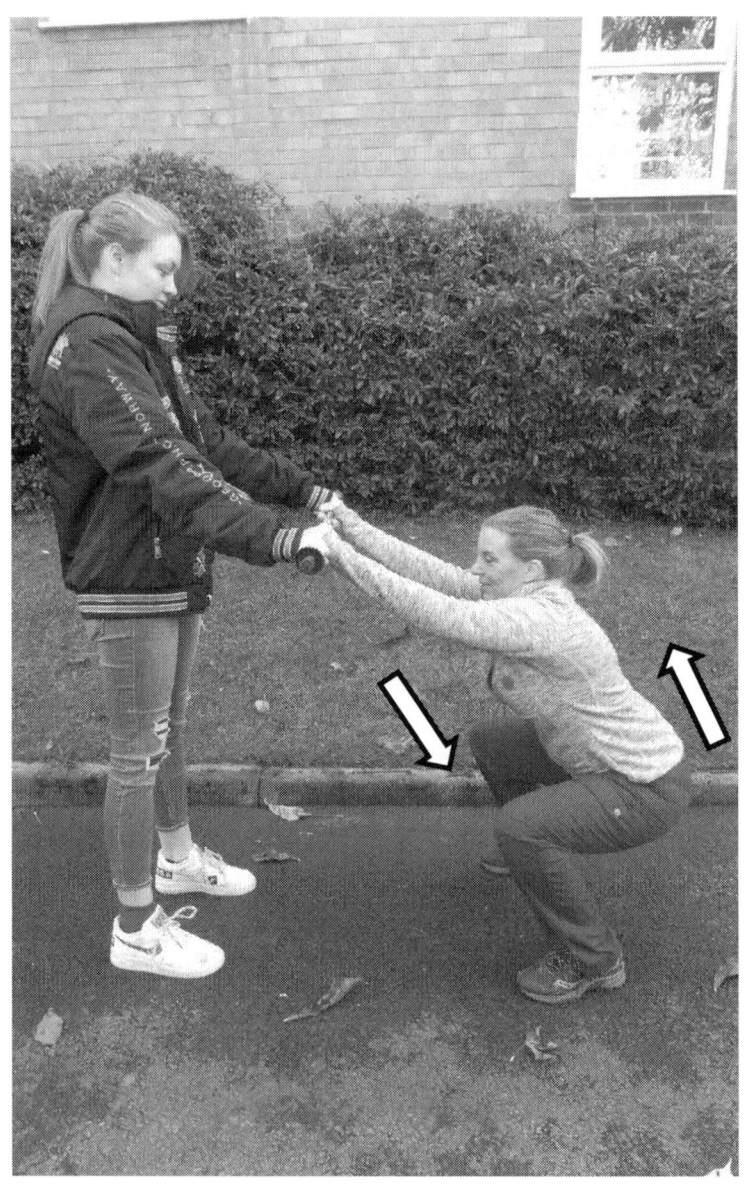

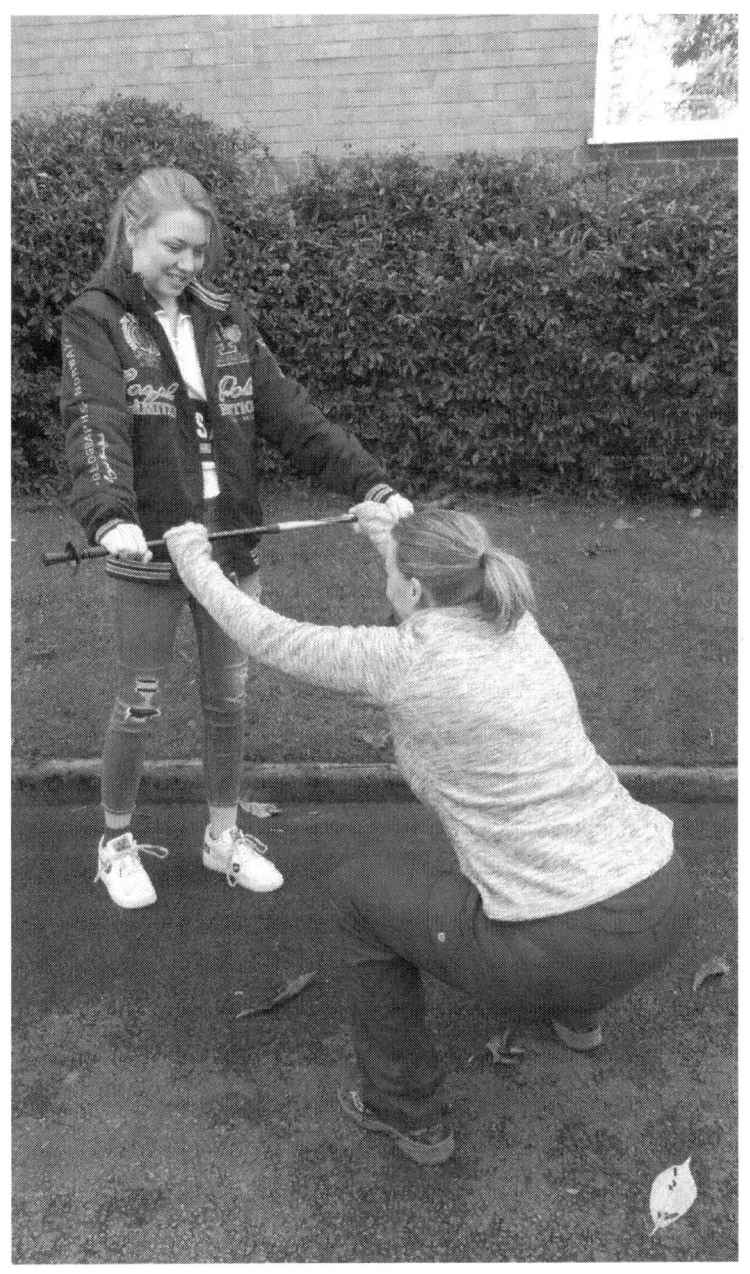

Legs – Thighs
Partner Pole Assisted-Resisted Squat

To perform this exercise the assisting partner stands behind the exercising partner at a medium to close distance. The exercising partner stands with their feet approximately shoulder-width apart and they hold the pole across their shoulders behind their neck.

The exercising partner bends the knees and assumes a squat position, ideally with the thighs parallel to the floor or as near to that as possible. As they squat they keep their back straight and bend forward only from the hips. The squat position is then held to perform the exercise which primarily targets the thighs and buttocks.

Once in the deepest part of the squat position, the assisting partner can either offer balance and/or resistance reduction by applying gentle pressure to slightly lift the pole. Alternatively, if the exercising partner is already quite fit and strong, the assisting partner can apply gentle resistance to add weight to the squat which will make the exercise more challenging.

Some people may either intentionally or inadvertently lean backward as they squat due to flexibility issues in their knees, ankles and hips. For this reason, the assisting partner must be aware of this possibility and brace their stance to accommodate for any shift in weight that may follow if their exercising partner does this.

Both partners must agree when to disengage from the exercise to prevent the other from suddenly losing balance and possibly even falling if one party stops the exercise abruptly for any reason.

The harder you engage the muscles, the more intense the exercise becomes, so always be sure to exercise at an intensity that best suits your individual ability. When you perform an isometric exercise never hold your breath. Always breathe deeply and naturally, which will be about 10 full breaths in and out at a rate of about 1 second per full breath. Perform each exercise for no less than 7 seconds, and for no longer than 10.

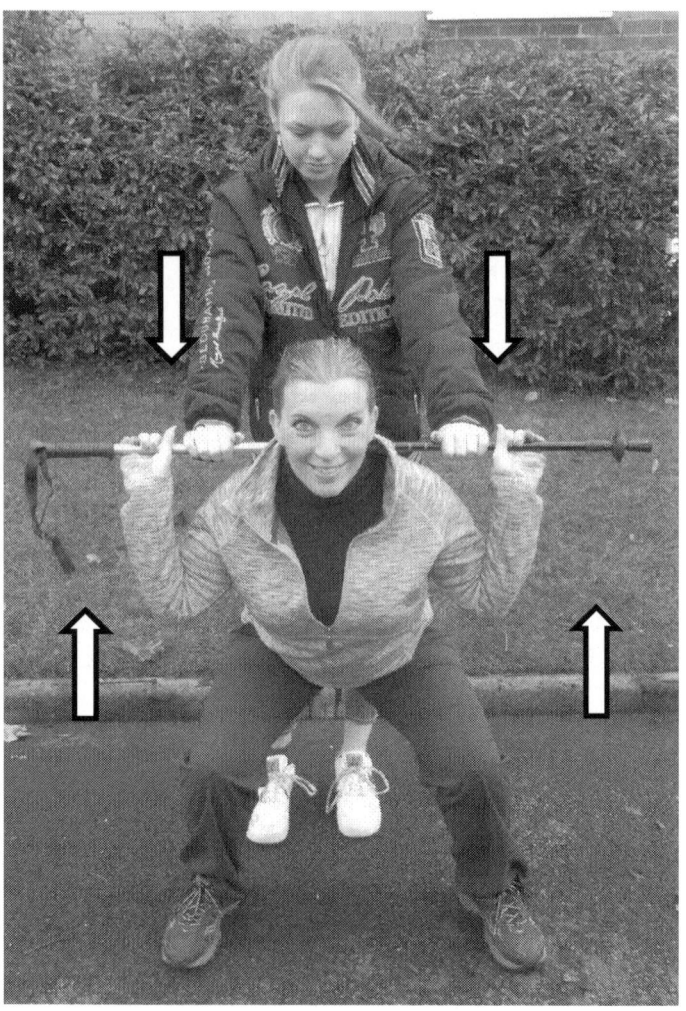

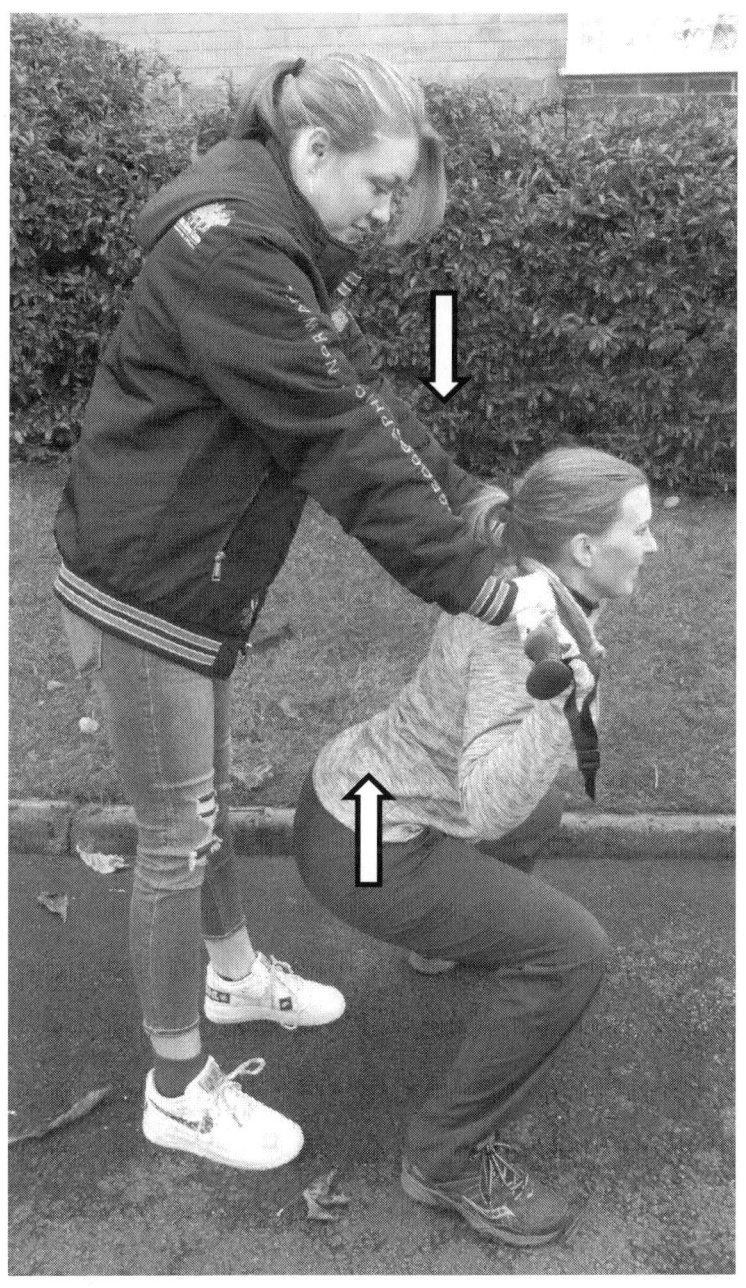

Shoulders - Partner Pole Resisted Front Arm Raise

To perform this exercise both partners stand upright, face to face at approximately arm's length from each other. The pole is held horizontally at somewhere between the exercising partner's waist height, and the highest point is the height of the exercising partner's shoulders.

The assisting partner grips the pole with a hand position that is slightly less than shoulder-width apart, and the exercising partner grips the pole at about shoulder-width apart. Both partners have outstretched arms with the elbows slightly bent and locked in that slightly bent position so they will not move during the exercise.

The exercising partner then applies pressure using the shoulder muscles to try and raise the arms forward and upwards. This is resisted by the assisting partner until the static exercise position is reached. This is when the exercise begins and exercises the shoulder muscles.

Both partners must agree when to disengage from the exercise to prevent the other from suddenly losing balance and possibly even falling if one party stops the exercise abruptly for any reason.

The harder you engage the muscles, the more intense the exercise becomes, so always be sure to exercise at an intensity that best suits your individual ability. When you perform an isometric exercise never hold your breath. Always breathe deeply and naturally, which will be about 10 full breaths in and out at a rate of about 1 second per full breath. Perform each exercise for no less than 7 seconds, and for no longer than 10.

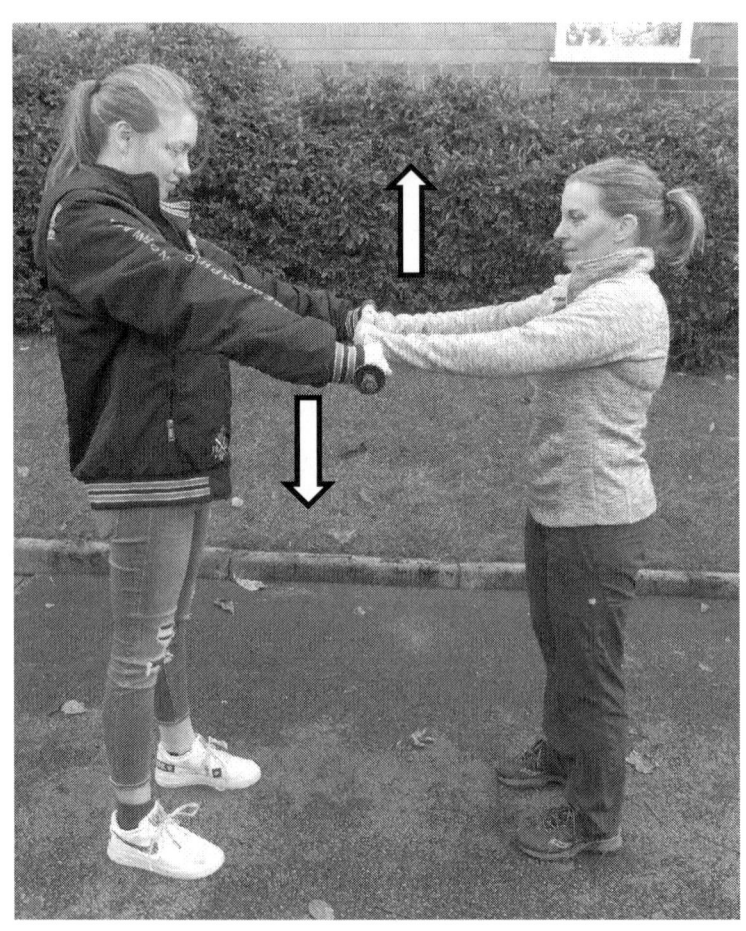

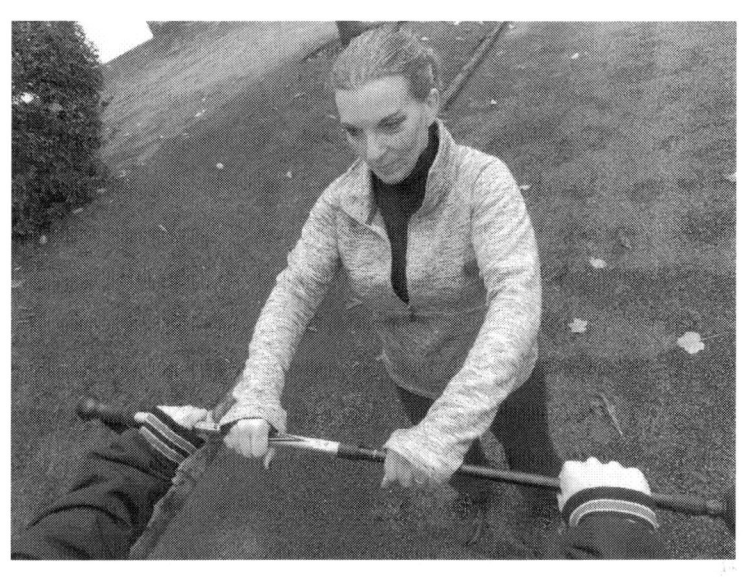

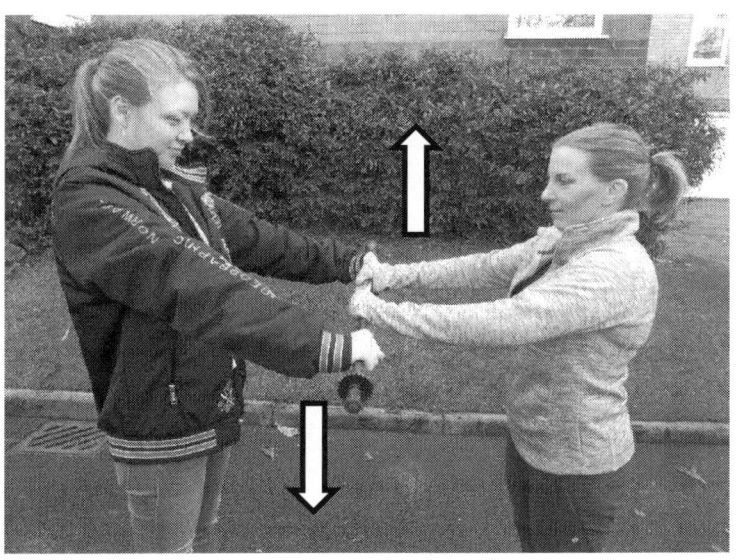

Shoulders - Partner Resisted Lateral Raise

To perform this exercise both partners stand upright with the assistant partner standing close behind the exercising partner. The exercising partner has both arms down but locked with the elbows in a slightly bent position with the palms facing the body. They then raise both of their arms sideways ensuring the palms of the hands face the body as they do so until they reach a mid-point position between waist and shoulder level.

At this point, the assisting partner places their hands on the upper forearms of the exercising partner to prevent the exercising partner's arms from raising further. They also to provide downward resistance as if attempting to force the exercising partner's arms back down to the starting position at waist height. This is when the exercise begins and exercises the shoulder muscles.

Both partners must agree when to disengage from the exercise to prevent the other from suddenly losing balance and possibly even falling if one party stops the exercise abruptly for any reason.

The harder you engage the muscles, the more intense the exercise becomes, so always be sure to exercise at an intensity that best suits your individual ability.

When you perform an isometric exercise never hold your breath. Always breathe deeply and naturally, which will be about 10 full breaths in and out at a rate of about 1 second per full breath. Perform each exercise for no less than 7 seconds, and for no longer than 10.

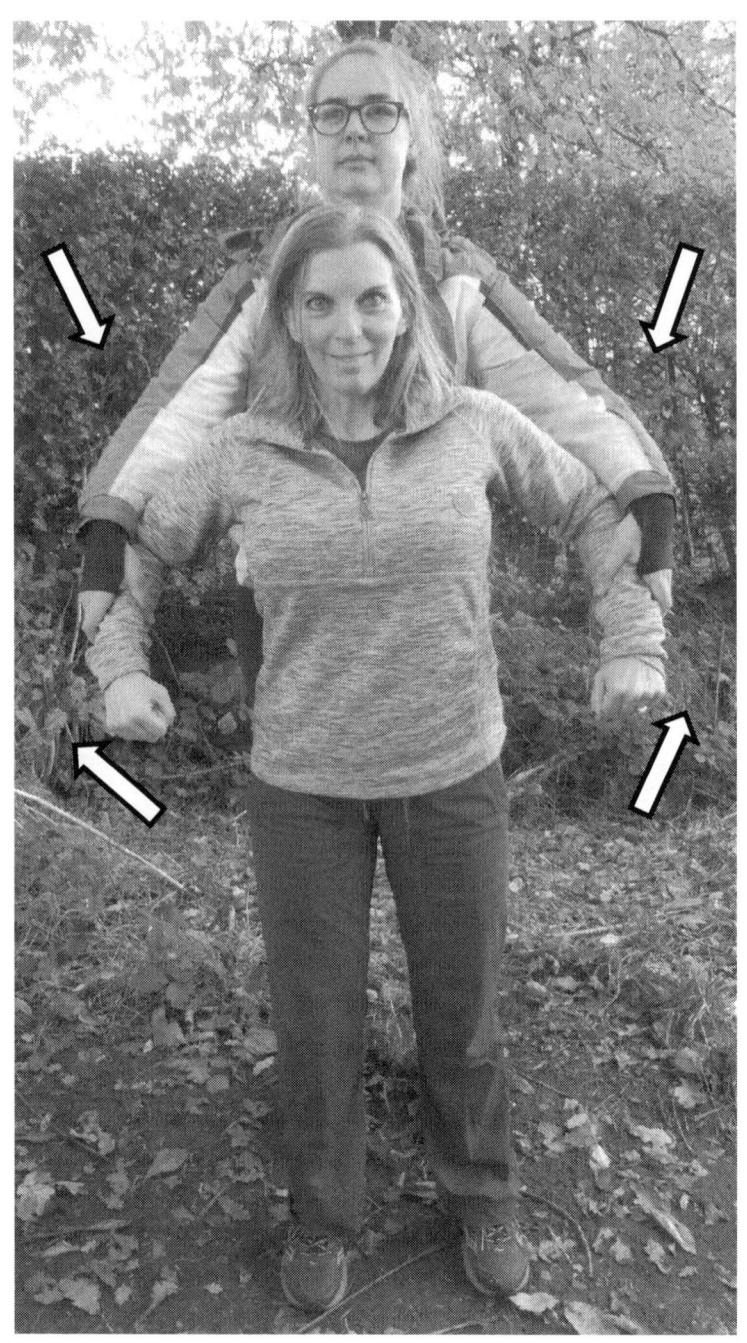

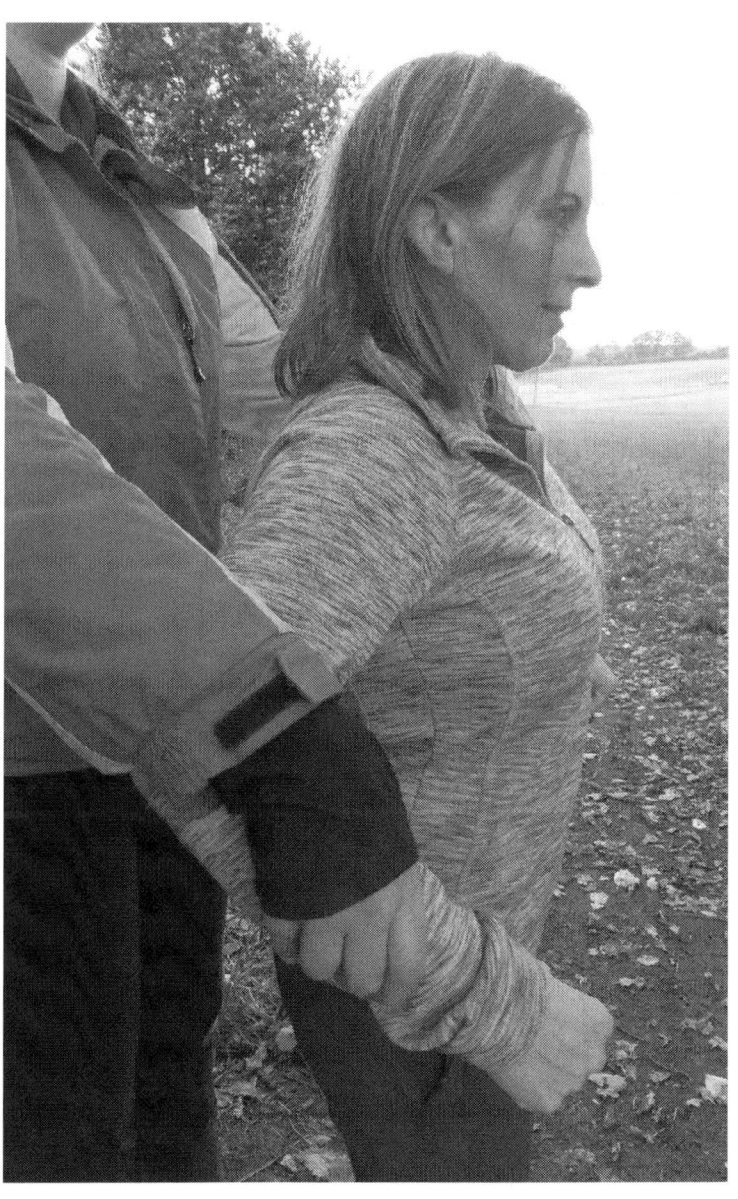

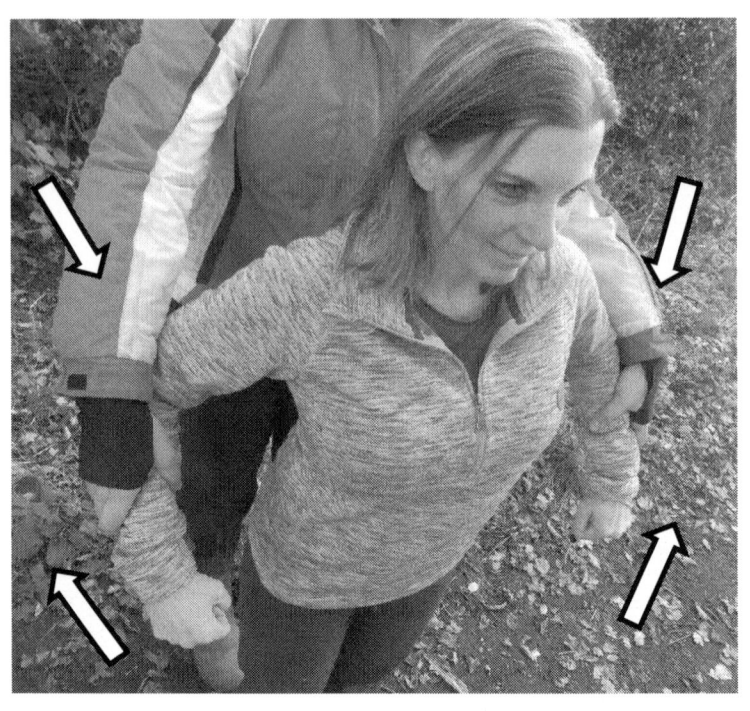

Shoulders
Partner Pole Resisted Press Behind Neck

To perform this exercise both partners stand upright with the assistant partner standing close behind the exercising partner.

The exercising partner stands with their feet approximately shoulder-width apart as they hold a pole above their head with their hands wider than shoulder-width apart. They should be wide enough apart so that at the mid-point position their bent arms should be at approximately 90-degrees.

In this position, the exercising partner applies force to press both inwards and slightly upwards at the same time. To oppose this, the assisting partner holds the pole evenly and uses their muscle power and bodyweight to resist the upward motion of the pole. This will target the entire shoulder, upper back and neck region.

Both partners must agree when to disengage from the exercise to prevent the other from suddenly losing balance and possibly even falling if one party stops the exercise abruptly for any reason.

The harder you engage the muscles, the more intense the exercise becomes, so always be sure to exercise at an intensity that best suits your individual ability. When you perform an isometric exercise never hold your breath.

Always breathe deeply and naturally, which will be about 10 full breaths in and out at a rate of about 1 second per full breath. Perform each exercise for no less than 7 seconds, and for no longer than 10.

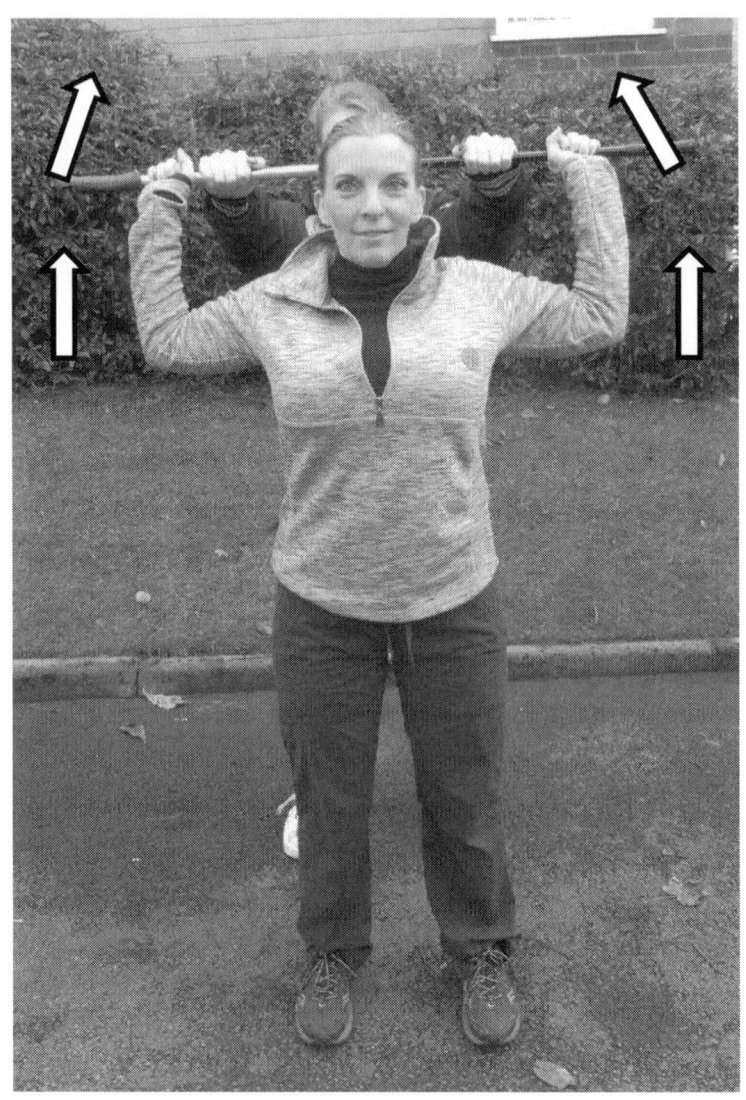

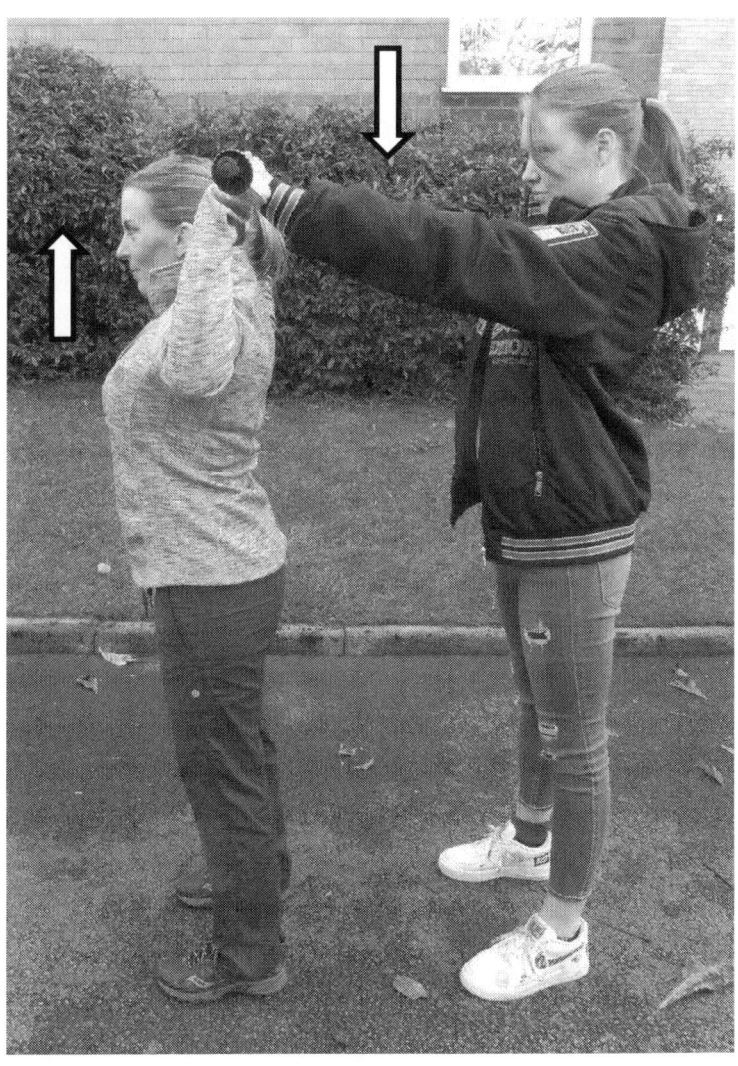

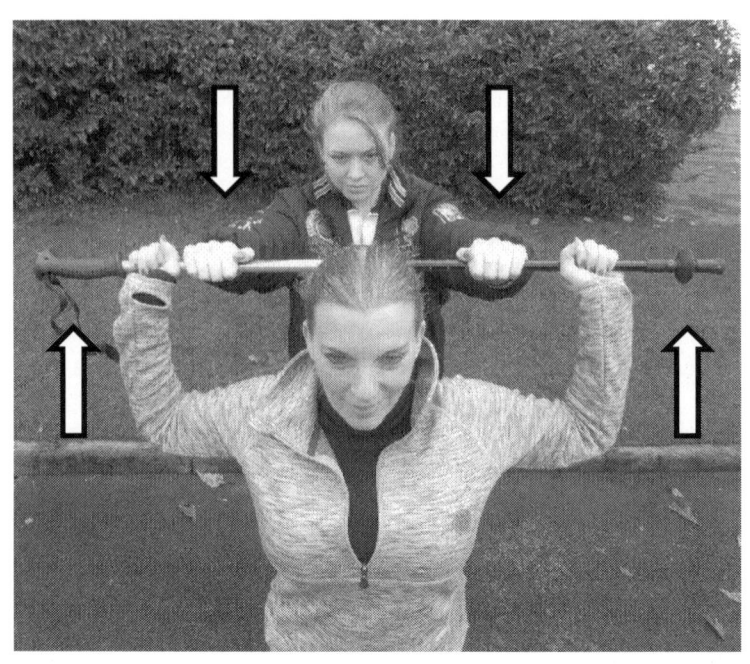

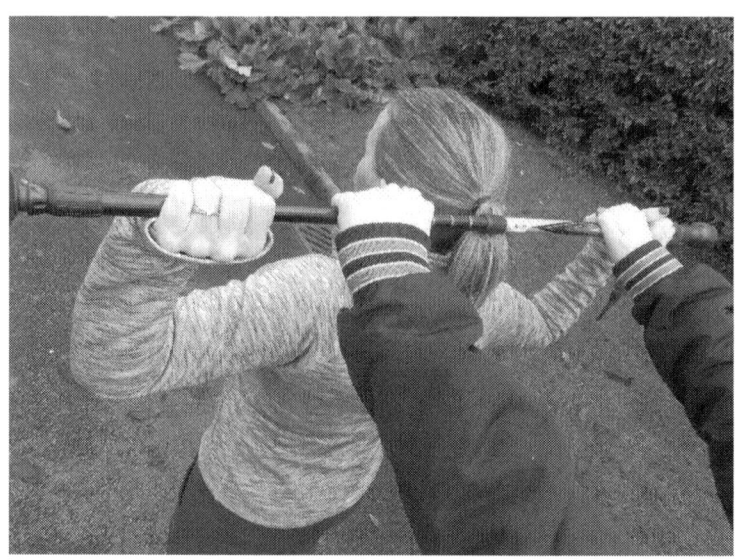

Shoulders - Partner Pole Resisted Front Press

To perform this exercise both partners stand upright close together and facing each other. The exercising partner stands with their feet approximately shoulder-width apart as they hold a pole in front of them horizontally at shoulder height, just about at chin level.

Their hands should be positioned wider than shoulder-width apart, and wide enough apart so that at the mid-point position their bent arms should be at approximately 90-degrees.

To oppose this, the assisting partner holds the pole evenly and in a similar position to allow them to use their muscle power and bodyweight to resist the upward motion of the pole. This will target the entire shoulder, upper back and neck region for the exercising partner.

Both partners must agree when to disengage from the exercise to prevent the other from suddenly losing balance and possibly even falling if one party stops the exercise abruptly for any reason.

The harder you engage the muscles, the more intense the exercise becomes, so always be sure to exercise at an intensity that best suits your individual ability. When you perform an isometric exercise never hold your breath.

Always breathe deeply and naturally, which will be about 10 full breaths in and out at a rate of about 1 second per full breath. Perform each exercise for no less than 7 seconds, and for no longer than 10.

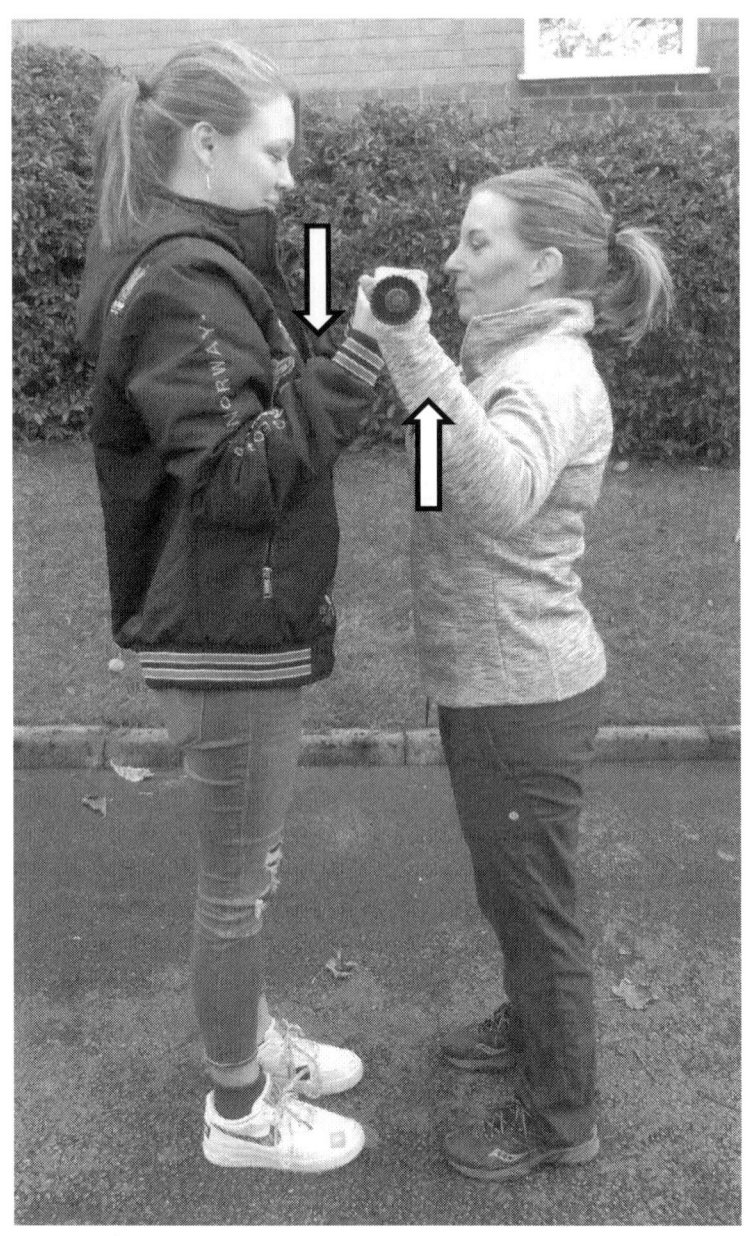

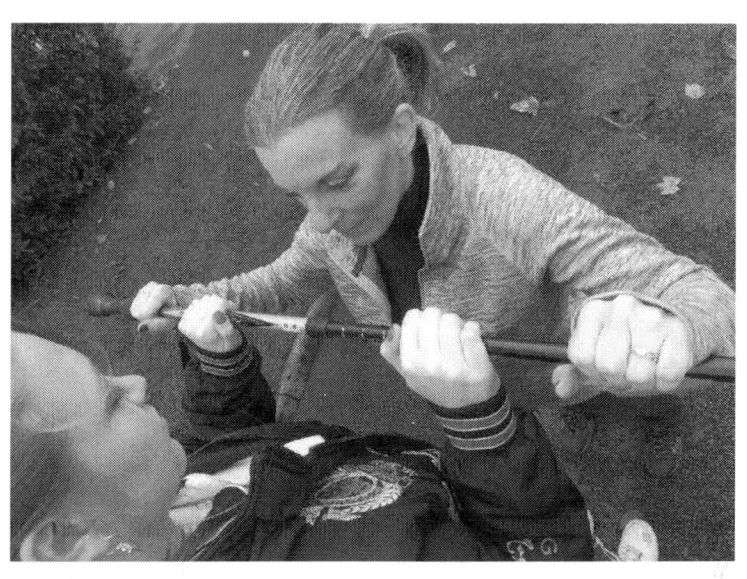

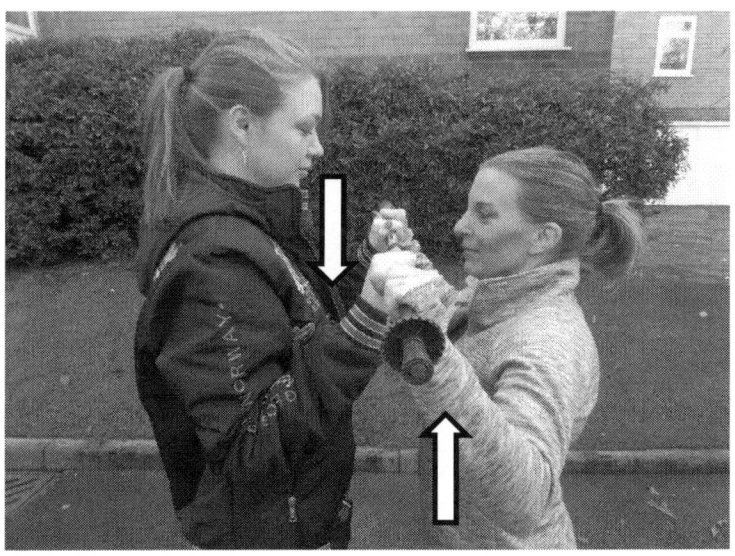

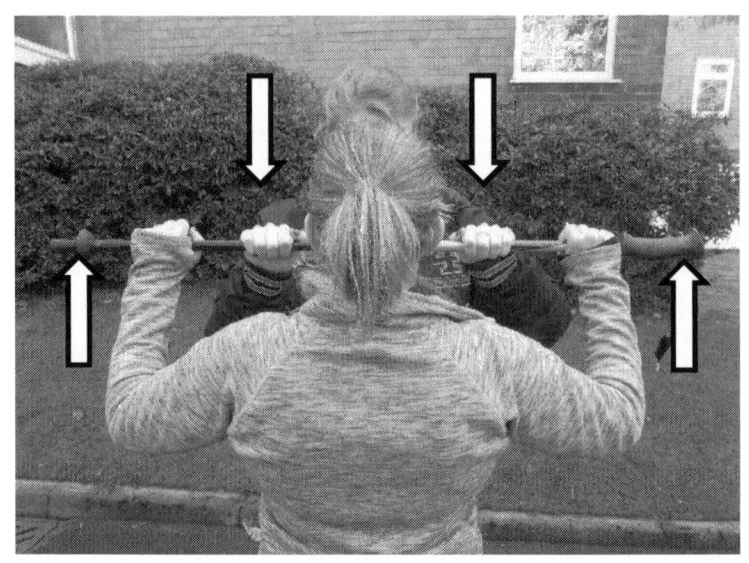

Shoulders - Partner Pole Resisted Upright Row

To perform this exercise both partners stand upright close together and facing each other. The exercising partner stands with their feet approximately shoulder-width apart as they hold a pole in front of them horizontally at waist height. Their hands should be positioned mid-point on the pole approximately slightly wider than thumbs-width apart and with their palms facing downwards.

To oppose this, the assisting partner holds the pole evenly and in a similar slightly wider handgrip position to allow them to use their muscle power and bodyweight to resist the upward motion of the pole.

The exercising partner keeps their arms and hands away from their body and applies force to raise the pole upwards leading the lifting action with their elbows moving forwards and upwards.

The assisting partner does not allow the pole to move up past the midpoint between the starting position and shoulder height, a point approximately at the height of their upper stomach and lower chest. This will target the entire shoulder, upper back and neck region for the exercising partner.

Both partners must agree when to disengage from the exercise to prevent the other from suddenly losing balance and possibly even falling if one party stops the exercise abruptly for any reason.

The harder you engage the muscles, the more intense the exercise becomes, so always be sure to exercise at an intensity that best suits your individual ability. When you perform an isometric exercise never hold your breath.

Always breathe deeply and naturally, which will be about 10 full breaths in and out at a rate of about 1 second per full breath. Perform each exercise for no less than 7 seconds, and for no longer than 10.

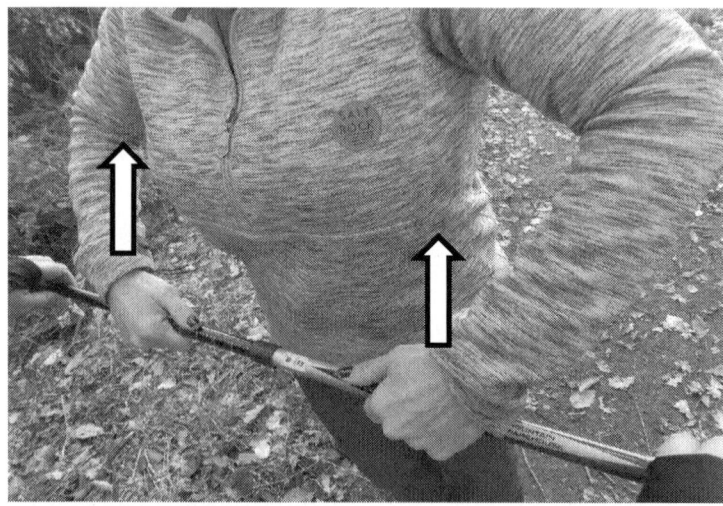

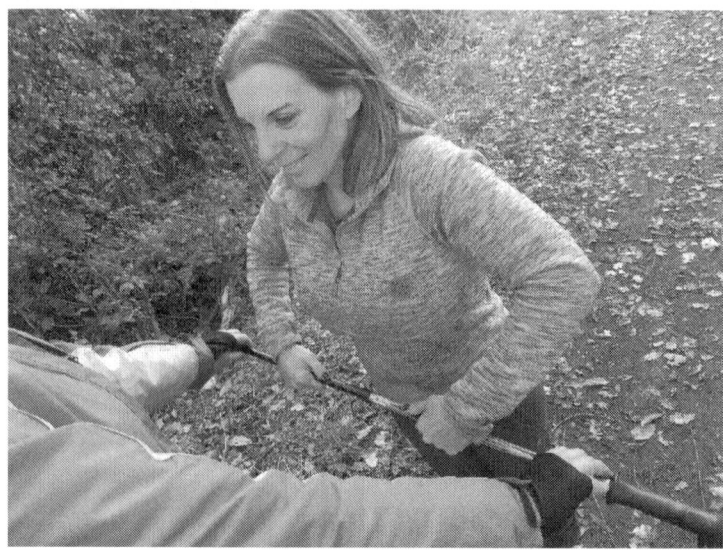

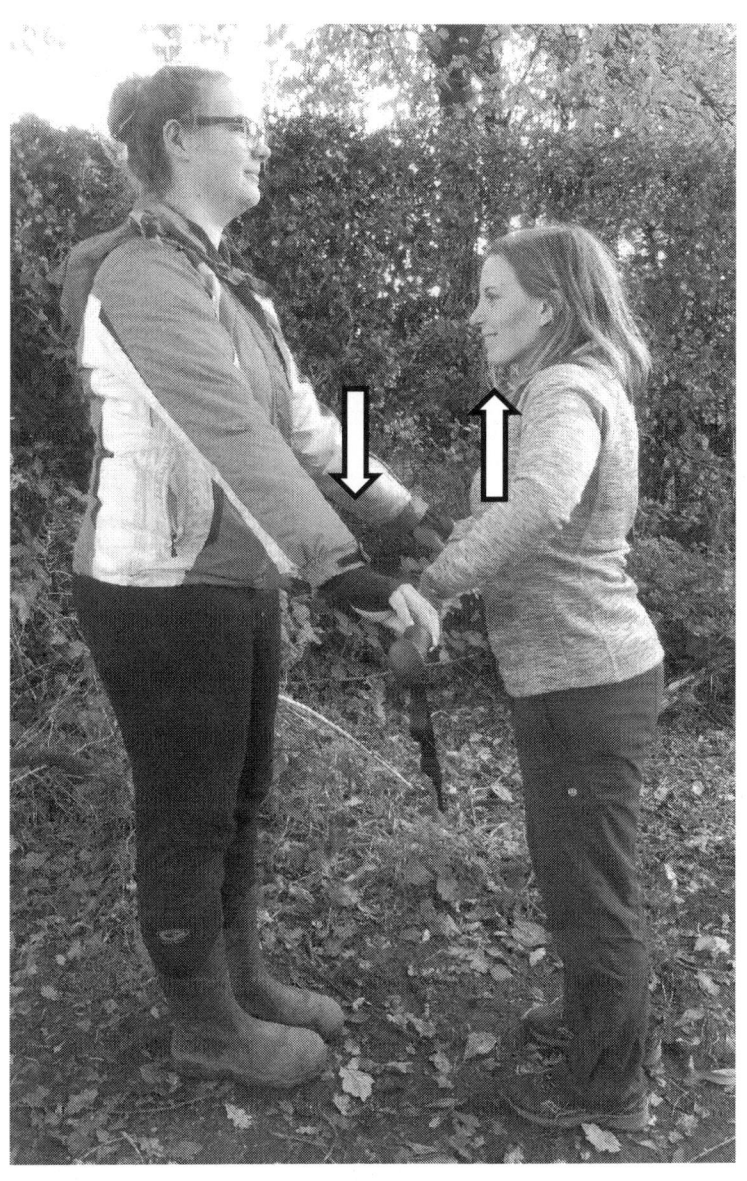

Chapter 7: Conclusion

Nordic Walking and Trekking are both excellent forms of exercise that can be enjoyed by people of almost all ages and almost all abilities. To many people, they are great ways to explore fascinating and hitherto unknown places. If walks are organised as a group activity then it becomes a fun-filled, informative, and friendly environment of likeminded people sharing their love of life, exploring and fitness together. Naturally, there are also many people who prefer the solace of walking as an individual. They love being alone and one with the wide-open spaces of the world. Or, they choose to share their frequently exhilarating exploration experiences with their life-partners.

No matter what kind of walking is preferred, be it Nordic Walking or traditional Trekking, the overall experience can be greatly enhanced by incorporating an isometric exercise routine at some point during the walk. Aside from the proven effectiveness of the exercise system, isometric exercise is quick, easy-to-perform, and an excellent way to exercise anywhere you choose. With simple, yet powerful isometrics, one can enjoy a total-body workout routine literally anywhere. For regular gym-users who for years have been caught in the "I can never be too far away from a gym" mental trap, this really is one of the most freeing experiences possible.

When we wrote our book called Fitness on the Move™ the exercises we selected to incorporate in it were the same ones we'd been performing ourselves on our world-wide travels over the years. We've enjoyed gym-quality total-body isometric exercise routines on while the move in some highly unusual places. Once I performed an isometric exercise routine with the cult moviemaker Cliff Twemlow on the deck of a ship in a storm on the Mediterranean sea as we travelled from Ibiza to Barcelona. Helen and I have performed total body isometric workout routines on beaches all over the world, from Cornwall to California, on mountainsides, and by lakes and lochs in Cumbria, Scotland, Iceland, and across North America and Canada. We've exercised effectively on long plane journeys without ever leaving our seat, as passengers in cars, on buses and on trains. Once, while we were waiting for the rest of our tour party we even had a "70 Second Difference™" isometric workout 2341 feet underground in the Soudan Mine, on the south shore of Lake Vermilion, in the Vermilion Mountain Range in Minnesota, USA.

Thanks to the isometric exercise system we've literally been able to exercise anywhere and everywhere we wanted to. One for the best things about it all has been that to perform a total body workout routine we typically needed no equipment or only the bare minimum that could easily fit into our pocket. After reading this book, you now know that you can perform a highly effective isometric exercise routine with nothing except your bare hands. However, by using what we call IIED's, or Improvised Isometric Exercise Devices such as climbing rope, martial arts or regular belts, Nordic Walking/Trekking poles, or the amazing Iso-Bow™, then you're carrying a powerful portable gymnasium with you wherever you go.

Now, you know how the isometric exercise system works you also know how all of the afore-mentioned IIED's can be used with great effect to deliver a powerful and efficient workout wherever you choose to perform one.

Isometric exercise isn't should be only thought of as something that should only to be performed while outdoors Nordic Walking or Trekking. By incorporating a regular isometric exercise routine into your daily schedule at home it will work wonders for your overall strength, fitness and body shape. Your new-found fitness and strength will bring many additional benefits along with it. It will make general daily tasks easier to perform, and for many, it will mean that they will perform better at their chosen sports or physical pastimes. Crucially for some, regular isometric exercise will greatly improve their overall mobility and performance when it comes to simply climbing stairs and standing up from a chair unaided. The fact is that whatever one does in life that is physical, being stronger and fitter always makes it easier and more fun to do. Let isometric exercise be your key to unleashing your full potential no matter what your current age or ability might be.

Many professional Nordic Walking and Trekking group leaders are recognising the value and effectiveness of isometric exercise for themselves and their clients. As such, they are choosing to become accredited isometric exercise instructors through TWiEA, The World Isometric Exercise Association. This enables them to deliver safe, effective and enhanced exercise coaching anywhere they choose during walking breaks. We wish you every success in life and sincerely thank you for taking the time to read this book and to hopefully perform isometric exercises on a regular basis. For more information visit www.TWiEA.com

www.MajorVision.com

Isometric Exercises for Nordic Walking and Trekking™ - Part 1. Exercises for Individuals

This book has been approved by **TWiEA** – The World Isometric Exercise Association (www.TWiEA.com).

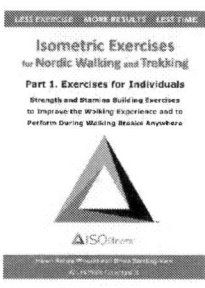

Strength and Stamina Building Exercises to Improve the Walking Experience and to Perform During Walking Breaks Anywhere. Nordic Walking and Trekking are two of the most popular forms of outdoor exercise that are available to almost anyone of almost any age or ability. Now, more Nordic Walkers and Trekkers than ever before are performing powerful and proven isometric exercise routines to exercise their whole body with gym-quality workout sessions during scheduled walk breaks in almost any location they choose. This book, Part 1., is an exercise resource guide of isometric exercises that can be performed as an individual, either outdoors or at home, and without the need for a buddy. Part 2. is an excellent resource guide of exercises to be performed in partnered pairs, with a walking buddy.

The 70 Second Difference™ - The Politically Incorrect,

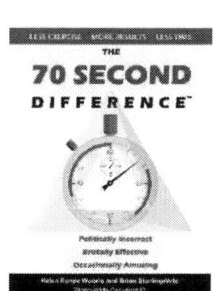

Occasionally Amusing, and Brutally Effective Guide to Strength, Fitness and Better Health

This book has been approved by **TWiEA** – The World Isometric Exercise Association (www.TWiEA.com).

This is a science-based no-nonsense guide that tells it straight about the most efficient ways to exercise, build muscle, get strong and how your deliberate lifestyle choices directly affect your body weight, overall health, fitness, strength and body shape. It also tells you how much protein you really need, and the dangers associated with dairy and animal-based products and meat. Lack of time is typically the enemy of fitness and regular exercise routines, however, just 70 seconds a day of focussed science-based exercise can solve the problem. Recommended Equipment: 2 x Iso-Bows®

The ISOmetric Bible™ - Exercise Anywhere with Scientifically Proven Isometrics

This book has been approved by **TWiEA** – The World Isometric Exercise Association (www.TWiEA.com).

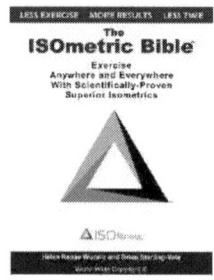

At 335 pages, the ISOmetric Bible™ is one of the most complete, scientific, practical, and user-friendly books on isometrics that's ever been written. Isometrics are proven by science to grow muscle and strength faster and more efficiently than any other exercise system. However, isometrics are also one of the most misunderstood forms of exercise, even by fitness professionals. An isometric exercise routine takes only minutes each day and can be performed anywhere you choose, on a plane, in a car, or even while you're at work. You don't need any special equipment to get a great total-body workout and the book shows you how to use easy to find everyday objects such as walking poles, broom handles, rope and towels to exercise with. Recommended Equipment: 2 x Iso-Bows®, some climbing rope and a towel.

TRISOmetrics™ - Advanced Science-Based High-Intensity Strength and Muscle Building

This book has been approved by **TWiEA** – The World Isometric Exercise Association (www.TWiEA.com).

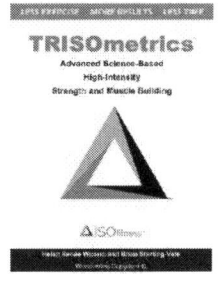

TRISOmetrics™ is an advanced, science-based high-intensity exercise system which combines 3 scientifically proven exercise techniques into a powerful new exercise system. It can be performed with or without equipment, making it ideal for use at home or when travelling. It can also be used as part of a gym-based heavy exercise routine; the choice is yours. It focusses on precision and quality in each exercise you perform combined with high-intensity to engage the maximum number of muscle fibres which keeps exercise sessions short, infrequent and highly effective. The system is ideal for people who don't confuse activity with accomplishment. Recommended Equipment: 2 x Iso-Bows®, climbing rope and a towel. It can also be performed with the Bullworker®, Steel Bow®, Bow Extension®, Iso-Gym® or similar and with all gym-based exercise equipment.

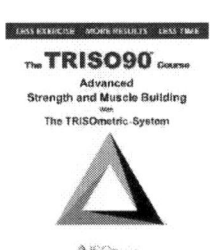

The TRISO90™ Course – Advanced Strength and Muscle Building with The TRISOmetrics™ System

This book has been approved by **TWiEA** – The World Isometric Exercise Association (www.TWiEA.com).

The TRISO90™ Course is a 534-page 90-day/12-week step-by-step advanced bodybuilding and strength-building exercise course based on the TRISOmetrics™ exercise system. The TRISOmetric™ exercise system consists of three proven science-based exercise principles which when combined, form this highly advanced high-intensity exercise technique. It is a highly advanced pure strength and muscle building course making it ideal for the natural bodybuilder or for anyone who wants to get into the best shape possible in the minimum amount of time, with or without equipment. Equipment: 2 x Iso-Bows®, dipping handles, some climbing rope and a towel.

The ISO90™ Course – The 12-Week/90-Day Shape-up and Get Strong Course

This book has been approved by **TWiEA** – The World Isometric Exercise Association (www.TWiEA.com).

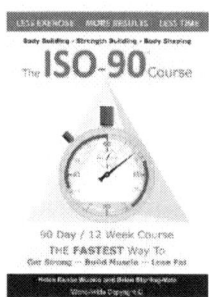

The ISO90™ Course is a comprehensive and complete step by step 90-day/12-week step-by-step isometric body shaping, bodybuilding and functional strength building course. It is ideal for both beginners and advanced trainers because your natural Adaptive Response™ mechanism means that whatever intensity you apply at whatever level you're at gives everyone roughly the same percentage of improvement. Required Equipment: 2 x Iso-Bows® available on Amazon or from Bullworker.com

Workout at Work™ - Exercise at Work Without Anyone Even Knowing What You're Doing!

This book has been approved by **TWiEA** – The World Isometric Exercise Association (www.TWiEA.com).

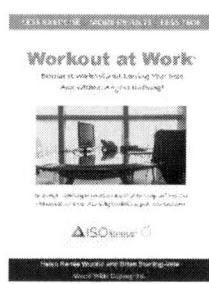

Time is the #1 reason why people don't exercise. The average person spends over 10 years of their life at work over an average 45 year working life, which can mean sitting at a desk for 10-years! There is never enough time to spare in modern life and exercising the traditional way in a gym 3-days a week, will consume a further 4.27 years. With proven isometric exercise, you can exercise effectively at work and even a complete beginner can benefit as much as an advanced athlete, all without ever leaving your desk. By performing just one simple 7-second high-intensity exercise every 30 minutes while sitting at your desk at the end of a 9-hour working day you'll have performed a powerful total-body 18-20 exercise routine. In exchange for just 126 seconds a day you'll feel better, be healthier, fitter, stronger, build more muscle and have more spare time to enjoy with family and friends. Your boss won't complain either because in exchange for just 126 seconds from work you'll be up to 30% more efficient at your job. Required Equipment: 2 x Iso-Bows® available on Amazon or from Bullworker.com

Fitness on the Move™ - Enjoy Gym-Quality Workout Sessions ANYWHERE!

This book has been approved by **TWiEA** – The World Isometric Exercise Association (www.TWiEA.com).

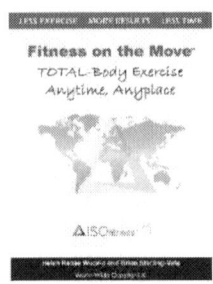

While travelling away from home for business or pleasure you can maintain your workout schedule if you're a beginner or advanced professional athlete. We've tested the Fitness on the Move™ system as passengers in cars, on trains, in airline seats, on mountainsides, on beaches, and once even on the deck of a ship in a storm. The Fitness on the Move™ system allows a full-body workout in the smallest space humanly possible thanks to our Zero Footprint Workout™ concept. If there is enough space to either sit down or stand upright, then you can perform a total-body exercise routine. Required Equipment: 2 x Iso-Bows® available on Amazon or from Bullworker.com

The Bullworker Bible™ The Ultimate Science-Based Guide to The Classic Personal Multi-Gym

This book has been approved by **TWiEA** – The World Isometric Exercise Association (www.TWiEA.com).

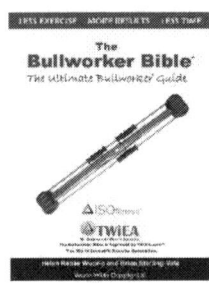

The Bullworker Bible™ is the definitive resource guide for all Bullworker® users, and it's the companion book for The Bullworker 90™ Course. The Bullworker Bible™ is approved by the makers, and distributors of The Bullworker®, at Bullworker.com. It is the complete science-based user-friendly guide of how the Bullworker® should be used properly to deliver maximum results. The Bullworker Bible™ gives you all the information that you need to know about repetition-compression and speed control, correct breathing techniques, how Hooke's Law of physics applies to The Bullworker®, and about correct biomechanics to deliver the best results. The Bullworker Bible™ is also the essential guide for all users of the Steel Bow®, Bullworker X5, Bully Extreme, ISO 7x, and the Bullworker X7. Required Equipment: Bullworker® Classic, or a similar. Recommended Additional Equipment: Steel Bow®, Bow Extension®, 2 x Iso-Bows®, and Bow Extension®.

The Bullworker 90™ Course – The Ultimate Science-Based 12-Week/90-Day Get strong and Grow Muscle Course Using the Classic Personal Multi-Gym

This book has been approved by **TWiEA** – The World Isometric Exercise Association (www.TWiEA.com).

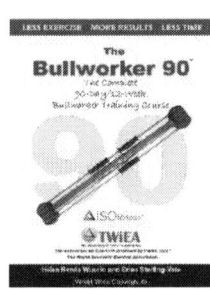

The Bullworker 90™ Course is a 400+ page 90-day/12-week step-by-step course for all Bullworker® users, and it's the companion book to The Bullworker Bible. Both books are approved by the makers of The Bullworker®. New exercises are added almost every week, with complete routine changes every two weeks. Each week has a detailed note section, together with suggestions about exercise days, and rest times etc. This means that you know exactly what to do, and when to do it. The Bullworker 90™ Course can be used with the Bullworker® Classic, the Steel Bow®, the Bullworker X5, the Bully Extreme, the ISO 7x, and the Bullworker X7. The Bullworker 90™ Course also contains alternative/extra exercises using the Iso-Bow® and the Bow Extension® to increase the range and effectiveness of The Bullworker®.

150

Required Equipment: A Bullworker® Classic, or a similar device. Recommended Equipment: Steel Bow®, Bow Extension® kit, 2 x Iso-Bows®.

The Bullworker Compendium™ - The Bullworker Bible™ and The Bullworker90™ Course Combined

This book has been approved by **TWiEA** – The World Isometric Exercise Association (www.TWiEA.com).

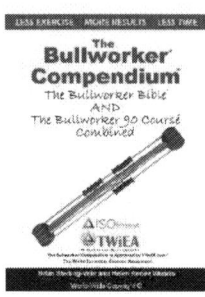

At over 575 pages The Bullworker Compendium™ is the combination of both The Bullworker Bible™ and The Bullworker 90™ Course in a single huge book.   To save printing costs the only thing we've eliminated are duplicated sections, everything else remains the same.   This way we're able to offer both books in one for less than the combined price of the two other books.   The Bullworker Compendium™ starts with The Bullworker Bible™, and at the end of that, it progresses seamlessly into The Bullworker 90™ Course.

Isometric Power Exercises for Martial Arts™ - Build Superior Strength, Muscle and Martial Arts 'Firepower' Using the Proven System Bruce Lee Used

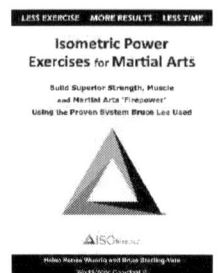

This book has been approved by TWiEA – The World Isometric Exercise Association (www.TWiEA.com).

Isometric exercise has been a part of almost every system of the martial arts ever devised. Even before isometrics were studied scientifically and modern

151

science-based training techniques were devised they have been taught and practised in one form or another for thousands of years. It was the great Bruce Lee and his love of isometric exercise who ensured that they would forevermore be famously linked to all types of martial arts training. This book contains a valuable resource of practical isometric exercises to build serious strength, muscle and martial arts 'firepower' needed by all types of martial artists. More importantly, isometric exercise builds solid, hard, practical muscle and not the bodybuilder type of bulk that would seriously restrict a martial artist. The author is recognised as one of the leading authorities on isometric exercise and has practised several different styles of martial arts for almost 50-years. Among his many awards and accolades, he is a WKA 8th Degree Black Belt and a recipient of a WKA Lifetime Achievement Award.

The Doorway to Strength™ - Turn a Door into a Strength-Building Multigym

This book has been approved by **TWiEA** — The World Isometric Exercise Association (www.TWiEA.com).

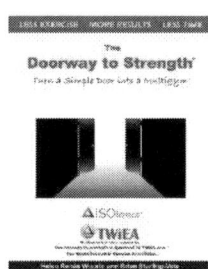

The Doorway to Strength™ shows how a simple door, doorway, and doorframe can be used to create a multi-gym of exercises using the amazing Iso-Bow® exerciser. It demonstrates how to perform a host of powerful and effective isometric exercises such as the door leg press and shoulder power push, together with many other exercises to work all the major body parts. Required Extra Equipment: 2 x Iso-

Bows® (preferably 4), a solid door and frame, and a door wedge/stop.

The Sixty Second ASS Workout™ - The Ultimate 60-Second Workout to Shape, Tone, Lift and Give You the Backside You've Always Wanted

This book has been approved by **TWiEA** – The World Isometric Exercise Association (www.TWiEA.com).

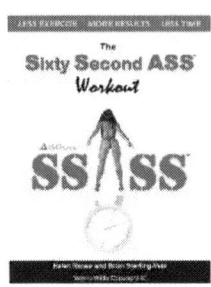

The Sixty Second ASS Workout™, or SSASS™ workout, is the fastest and most effective "ass" workout ever devised. Based on the scientifically proven principles of advanced isometric exercise, the SSASS™ workout is a no-nonsense time-efficient workout that does everything you need to make your ass tight, firm, shapely and strong. No more time-wasting workouts where you twist, shake, wiggle around, kick your legs, or dance around for 30 minutes which are fun but never deliver the results you want. Everyone has 60 seconds of time to spare, even on the busiest day, so, you're just 60 seconds a day from having a great ass. Required Equipment: 2 x Iso-Bows available on Amazon or from Bullworker.com

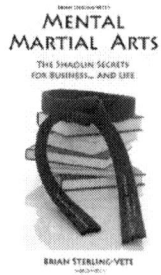

Mental Martial Arts™ - intellectual Life and Business Combat Skills
Brian Sterling-Vete's Mental Martial Arts is a system of intellectual life-combat skills using the tactics and principles of the physical martial arts. All interaction in life, in business, and when

communicating with others is simply an exchange of energy, power and influence. Each party is always exerting maximum influence over the other to gain the outcome they prefer. The more powerful and persuasive will usually win unless the apparently 'weaker' person is trained in the Mental Martial Arts. You can learn how to verbally, intellectually, and emotionally guide, channel and redirect the energy of others, even powerful people and large organisations to more frequently achieve the outcome that you desire in life and business. It also contains a section about how to handle a potentially hostile media in the event of a crisis where the experience Brian gained in over a decade with BBC TV News and a lifetime in the martial arts can help you and your organisation stay Media Safe. www.mentalmartialarts.tv

Tuxedo Warriors™

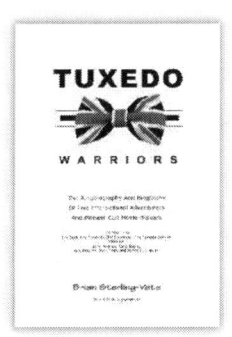

Tuxedo Warriors is the companion book to both The Tuxedo Warrior book and the movie. These books are the biography and autobiography of the iconic cult author, composer, moviemaker Cliff Twemlow. The original book ended at the beginning of what has been called by many 'the Golden Age' of Video Cinematography which Cliff Twemlow inspired. Tuxedo Warriors continues the story from the point when Cliff's original book finishes, and it is the most complete biography of Cliff Twemlow ever written. It's also the autobiography Brian Sterling-Vete who played a central role in this unique, entertaining and true story of two 'Renaissance-Men' and their adventures as guerrilla moviemakers.

The Tuxedo Warrior™ by Cliff Twemlow – Prologue and epilogue by Brian Sterling-Vete.

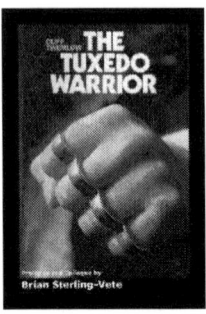

There are many ways in which a Doorman can gain respect. Numerous methods applied to the principal. In my profession, every available technique must be utilised, depending on the situation and circumstances. Would-be transgressors either move-off the premises quietly acknowledging your diplomatic approach. Or, the other alternative whereby physical persuasion must be exercised, which either quells their pugilistic desires or it triggers their aggressive instincts, turning the whole incident into a bloody and violent encounter. 'The Tuxedo Warrior,' pulls no punches in its brawling, savage, colourful, and entertaining exposure of society's nightlife activities.

The above is the original text from the rear cover of Cliff's book. Where Cliff's original book finishes, my own book 'Tuxedo Warriors' begins to complete Cliff's colourful life story. I'm honoured to be friends with Cliff's eldest son, Barry, and sincerely thank him for enabling this book and the others that Cliff wrote to be re-published.

The Pike™ by Cliff Twemlow – Prologue and epilogue by Brian Sterling-Vete.

ITS FIRST VICTIMS - A screeching swan... A fisherman overboard... A drunken woman...

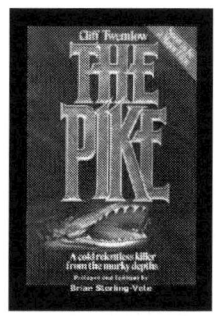

One by one, the mysterious killer in Lake Windermere claims its terrified victims. Tearing off limbs with its monstrous teeth, horribly mutilating bodies. Fear sweeps the peaceful holiday resort when experts identify the creature as a giant pike…. A hellish creature with the strength to rupture boats, and the anger to attack them. But for some, the terror becomes a bonanza—the traders who cater to the gathering crowds of ghouls on the shore. And, they will do anything to stop divers finding the creature. Meanwhile the ripples of bloodshed widen…. The Pike.

The above is the original text from the rear cover of Cliff's book which was to become a movie in the early 1980s starring Joan Collins.

The Beast of Kane™

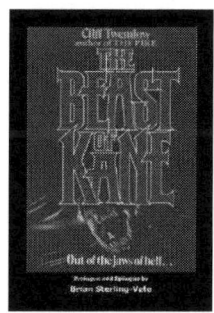

by Cliff Twemlow – Prologue and epilogue by Brian Sterling-Vete.

When the Gordon Family open their door to a stray Elkhound, they unwittingly welcome-in the forces of evil. For, according to the local priest, the huge dog is Satan himself, fulfilling an ancient prophecy. But, no one will believe this warning… Even when sheep – and wolves – are mysteriously slaughtered. Even when frenzied pets turn on their owners. Even when Emily Forrest is savagely eaten alive – the first of many human victims. As winter tightens its icy grip on the remote town of Kane, its unprotected people must face an unearthly terror.

The above is the original text from the rear cover of Cliff's book. This was the first of Cliff's books to be accepted by Hammer Film Studios to be made into a big-screen horror movie, along with Cliff's other book, The Pike.

The Haunting of Lilford Hall™ - The Birthplace of the United States as a Nation Haunted by the Man Behind The Pilgrim Fathers

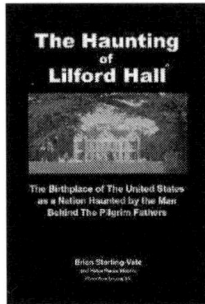

The Haunting of Lilford Hall is one of the most baffling cases ever recorded of paranormal activity experienced simultaneously by multiple people. Between 2012 and 2013, a team of 13 people came together to produce a historical TV documentary, not a paranormal investigation. The TV documentary was about the life of Robert Browne, the man who was behind The Pilgrim Fathers sailing on The Mayflower to settle the first civilian colony on the American continent. In fact, without Robert Browne, there may never have been the United States of America, at least not as we know it today. They experienced doors that refused to stay closed, they had debris thrown at them, they had a door silently ripped away from the hinges and doorframe while they were in the next room. There were even several recorded multi-witness apparitions of a man fitting Robert Browne's recorded description. It is believed by many that the ghost of Robert Browne, the "Grandfather" of the United States as a nation, still haunts Lilford Hall to this day.

- Robert Browne was the man who separated church from state in the reign of Queen Elizabeth 1st which is the underpinning of the United States.
- Robert Browne's words are written into the constitution of the United States.
- Robert Browne's direct descendent officially fired the first shot in the American war of independence.
- Robert Browne's beloved Lilford Hall estate was the home of President George Washington's Mother.
- Robert Browne's beloved Lilford Hall estate was the home of President Quincy Adams' family.

Paranormal Investigation - The Black Book of Scientific Ghost Hunting and How to Investigate Paranormal Phenomena™

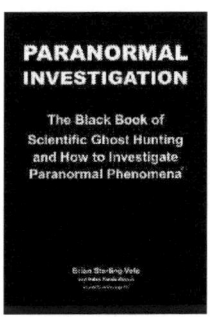

This book is ideal for those who are new to paranormal investigation and ghost hunting, and also for more experienced investigators who want to learn more about how to apply a critical-path scientific approach. It contains a special scientific critical path graphic page to work from when devising ghost hunting experiments and to help train team members. The book also contains a step-by-step guide to a complete paranormal investigation and important information about how to protect yourself from malevolent paranormal entities that can attack you. It also contains several example stories of previously untold paranormal events which have taken place, the ground-breaking Redwood Falls Minnesota UFO sighting, and about potentially paranormally active and potentially 'haunted' locations.

Being American Married to a Brit™ - An Amusing Guide for Anglo-American Couples Divided by a Common Language and Culture

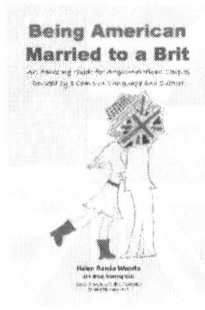

When I first started dating my British man, I never gave a second thought about differences in language and culture. Why would I? After all, we Americans speak English, or do we...? As dating quickly turned into being engaged to and then getting married to my British gentleman, I also found that our common language and culture was a quirky, eye-opening, and highly amusing roller-coaster ride. At times during the most basic every-day conversations, I'd be listening to his words with glazed eyes, wondering what on earth he was saying. It really was as if we were both speaking a completely different language, even though the words that comprised the language were the same. I very quickly learned so much more about the language I was supposed to have been taught at school, the commonalities, the differences, and the good old-fashioned belly-laughs about it all that still punctuate our married life to this day. So, I decided to write this book and dedicate it to all transatlantic couples who will regularly find themselves completely divided and confused by their common language and culture.

www.MajorVision.com

Printed in Germany
by Amazon Distribution
GmbH, Leipzig